The Beauty Buyble

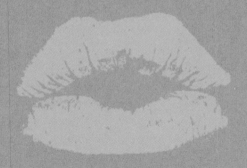

The Beauty Buyble

The Best Beauty Products

2007

Paula Conway & Maureen Regan

REGAN

An Imprint of HarperCollinsPublishers

HarperCollins books may be purchased for educational, business, or sales promotional use. For information please write: Special Markets Department, HarperCollins Publishers Inc., 10 East 53rd Street, New York, NY 10022.

FIRST EDITION

Designed by Kris Tobiassen

Printed on acid-free paper

Library of Congress Cataloging-in-Publication Data

Conway, Paula.
The beauty buyble : the best beauty products of 2007 / Paula Conway and Maureen Regan.
    p. cm.
    ISBN 10 0-06-117208-1
    ISBN 13 978-0-06-117208-3
    1. Beauty, Personal. 2. Cosmetics. 3. Consumer education. I. Regan, Maureen, 1961–
II. Title.

RA778.C66 2006
646.7'042—dc22

                                                    2006046518

06 07 08 09 10 RRD 10 9 8 7 6 5 4 3 2 1

We dedicate this book to girls of all ages.

Contents

PART III: Body

Foreword

This book contains hundreds of amazing products and quotes from some of the beauty industry's leading experts, many of them my friends. Having worked with celebrities, supermodels, and some of America's most influential movers and shakers, I can assure you that *The Beauty Buyble* is one of the most exciting and unique projects I've ever seen.

I have known Paula Conway as a beauty writer for several years, and one day she approached me to participate in a book project she was working on with Maureen Regan, *The Beauty Buyble*. When Paula asked me to write the foreword, I was beyond honored, and I'm so proud to be able to participate and share my intense passion for beauty with Paula and Maureen.

My father started his salon in Naples, Italy, back in 1955, and I've been passionate about hair since I was a young boy. When I started my first salon in New York City's legendary Plaza Hotel in 1997, my dream was to create hairstyles and products that reflected my extreme passion and desire to restore hair to its healthiest state with a combination of old-world Italian methods and pure ingredients. The Oscar Blandi hair care line was first launched in 2004, and we are especially proud to see how well the line is doing today as one of the leading prestige hair care lines in the country. In spring 2005 I opened a new luxury salon on Madison Avenue, and like everything else in my hair care domain, it truly reflects my Italian heritage.

Beauty is for everyone, and every woman has the right to be and feel beautiful. I hope that you will enjoy your *Beauty Buyble*. A great deal of passion has gone into this book, and in passion lies beauty.

Oscar Blandi

Introduction

Tormented by mascara that clumps? Driven witless with lipstick that's gone in an hour? Whipsawed with confusion over finding the right blow-dryer? Honey, look no further, *The Beauty Buyble* has arrived!

Call us the Nader's Raiders of the beauty industry—this is a beauty shakedown! We plumped our lips, tweezed our eyebrows, sampled every false eyelash, polished our toes and fingernails what seemed like a thousand times, shampooed, conditioned, rinsed, and then started over again. We waxed, fluffed, brushed, smoothed, sprayed, spritzed, glossed, whitened, and moisturized until we emptied every bottle and squeezed every tube. Then, we talked to the experts who create the looks for magazine covers and red carpet events and make the celebrities look like, well, celebrities. And after all this, we blackmailed beauty editors everywhere for their opinions and coerced a huge posse of real women (including our husbands) until they couldn't stomach another lip balm. The pets were spared only because we don't believe in animal testing.

We organized all products into three price categories—High, Medium, and Low—and then added one more category if the price was truly Outrageous.

➤ Products in the HIGH category generally cost $20 or more, or are the more expensive products for the category.

➤ MEDIUM products generally fit into more mortal budgets, ranging from $10 to $20, and/or represent products in the mid-range of the category.

➤ LOW products generally are under $10 or among the least expensive range of products for the category.

➤ If the price is unmanageable for most budgets, it is deemed OUTRAGEOUS.

If the quality of one or two clearly stands out, regardless of category, we label them Authors' Picks. These are the products we love the most despite the votes from the experts. We also let you know which products we love, make us happy, give us warm fuzzy feelings, and which we use ourselves. Quality products are not just about how much they cost, and the best in a category can be a low-cost product. Also, if there is no really good quality product within a certain price category, there might not be a High, Medium, or Low product recommended. It's all about getting you the best in each category, and if there is no quality product in the class, we don't do you the disservice of telling you the best of what we think is a shabby lot.

So how did we set about choosing products for this book? Did we just sit around the veranda sipping margaritas, taking in pedicures, and soaking in backrubs from the pool boys while we discussed the merits of the various products? Unfortunately, no. Did we use a very scientific method of throwing all the names into a hat and picking three? Again, no, although it would have made our lives a lot easier and would have made writing this book a much faster process. No, we went to great lengths interviewing experts who want to be named, insiders who demand to remain anonymous, and our intrepid testing team of real women from coast to coast and even tested the products ourselves to find the standout.

So here you have it: the best beauty products for 2007. But before you begin, you must hold your mascara tube high, repeat and swear by *The Beauty Buyble* Ten Commandments:

1. This is THE *Beauty Buyble,* you shall have no other publications before it.

2. Be true to your own beauty; rely not on beauty counter makeovers for your look.

3. You shall not take Chanel's name in vain.

4. Remember the body and keep it moisturized daily.

5. Honor your roots; ¼ inch and get thee some color.

6. Never leave the house without wearing an SPF of 15 or greater.

7. Cheat not on your hairstylist or colorist—they always know.

8. You shall not use lipstick as rouge—you're not fooling anyone.

9. Cleanliness is next to godliness—never go to bed with your makeup on.

10. You shall not covet your best friend's *Beauty Buyble*; buy your own!

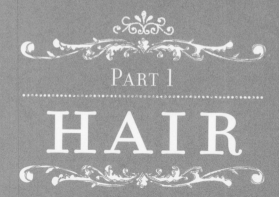

PART 1

HAIR

Hair is our crowning glory; it is the swirl at the top of the ice cream. It is the perch for our tiaras (and girls, who doesn't have her "princess tiara" tucked away in the back of the jewelry cabinet somewhere?), and tells everyone in an instant what kind of person you are. Few things reflect our personalities as clearly as hair, whether we are fun and frivolous, business-like and serious, or a real emotional mess (we all have those days from time to time). Nobody wants to be a flat, oily, messy frump—your hair needs proper care to keep you looking bouncy, stylish and carefree, yet in control.

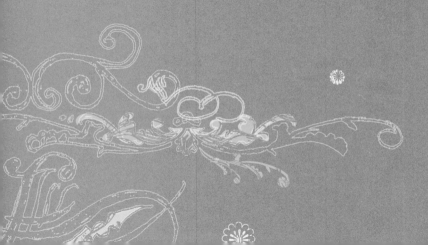

Shampoos

Selecting the right shampoo for your hair is like winning the Oscar. Your scalp will shout out "You like me, you really like me!" Without a good shampoo, your hair is just, well, poo. And nobody wants a head full of poo after all (our friends at Devachan will explain later in this chapter).

Eva Scrivo, Dove Hair Care Creative Consultant and New York City salon owner, offers the following tips on the subject of shampoo:

➤ Select the proper shampoo and conditioner for your hair type.

➤ For normal to oily hair, use a shampoo that thoroughly cleans the hair without stripping it. Brush normal to oily hair at least twice daily to distribute your hair's natural oils evenly along the hair shaft. Infrequent brushing can make your hair seem greasier than it really is, because oils stay deposited at your scalp.

➤ Fine, thin hair needs products that give it volume.

➤ Color-treated hair needs a shampoo and conditioner with a formula containing antioxidants and UV protectants to keep it from fading in the sun. Applying a styling product to finish your look also helps protect your hair from the sun and wind.

➤ Dry, damaged hair can rear its ugly head. If you're having trouble combing through your hair after washing it, then you need a moisturizing conditioner to smooth the breakage. Eva also recommends applying a weekly deep conditioning treatment immediately after washing. Wrap hair in a towel and let it sit for about twenty minutes to give hair a smooth, shiny appearance.

SHAMPOO QUICK TIP: Celebrity stylist Oscar Blandi, who creates stylish, sexy cuts for Ashley Judd, Sandra Bullock, and Reese Witherspoon, says, "You should always shampoo with medium temperature water; not too hot, not too cold. It may take a bit longer to rinse, but harsh temperatures will stress your hair out. Rinse with cool water to lock the product under the cuticle."

Dry Hair Shampoos

Your hair and scalp are as dry as the Sahara and you don't have a clue what to do. The answer, my friend, isn't blowin' in the wind. No, ma'am. Dry hair needs body, reinforcement, and protection.

HIGH Fresh Rice Shampoo ($24)
www.fresh.com

This shampoo gives super creamy lather a new definition—it's like a day spa for overworked, dry hair. Hair heaven is yours with this shampoo, oh, and the exotic Asian pear and persimmon are positively intoxicating scents for your head.

HIGH Shampoo di Jasmine Smoothing Shampoo ($20)
www.oscarblandi.com

This shampoo is ultragentle, moisture rich, and compatible for hair that is color-treated. The creamy texture contains avocado oil and nettle extract to add shine. This is a superb and highly recommended product for all hair types and is a savior for dry hair.

MEDIUM bc bonacure moisture shampoo from Schwarzkopf Professional ($12.50)
Fine salons or (800) 707-9997

If you can cast your mind back to a time when a woman couldn't get a loan, wasn't allowed to wear trousers to work and panty hose (then called tights) were required, even in the summer, because the office had a strict dress code for women, then you can understand why bc bonacure shampoo is so important today. Back then it was Breck or Body on Tap, shampoo that just cleansed the hair, a very minimal result to coincide with very limited potential in the office. Today, there are greater demands placed on women in the workforce, and thus greater demands on shampoo. This shampoo's technology actively targets dry areas, strengthens hair, and selectively repairs damage only where needed. It is a fact that with bc bonacure's moisture shampoo, life is more beautiful and the possibilities are endless.

LOW   L'Oreal VIVE Shampoo Nutri-Moisture ($3.99)
Mass retailers or www.drugstore.com

Takeaway is fine, and reheating is no problem, but don't ask us to spend a fortune on shampoo when we can afford this one and the results are on par with anything above it. It has a cashmere touch at a fraction of the price!

THE AUTHORS' PICK for this category—and this was a very close one, as all three picks are superb products—the L'Oreal VIVE shampoo because it consistently performs as it says it will and for the price, it's unbeatable. Another good thing is that you can purchase this product anywhere, and who hasn't forgotten their shampoo on a trip and then had to live with less-than-perfect hair because they couldn't find the right shampoo?

Oily Hair Shampoos

It feels like a mop that has just swabbed a public restroom, the heavy oily strands just weigh you down. The right shampoo can make you feel clean again, and give your hair some beautiful bounce and lightness.

HIGH   Phytopanama Mild Shampoo ($20)
Fine salons or www.sephora.com

Maureen:

On this sunny morning at the Canyon Ranch spa outside of Tucson, Arizona, I find myself stuck with an unusual dilemma: my hair is oily out here. As I plowed through another gallon of fruit-flavored water, an unsettling truth occurred to me. I haven't yet found the right shampoo for oily hair. We need to put our brains through some cardio, Maureen—help!
—Paula

Paula:

Don't fret. Upon receiving your e-mail I immediately gathered our hair panel for an impromptu conference call. It's unanimous. The Phytopanama is extremely mild, and this frequent-use shampoo contains 65 percent panama wood to cleanse, while respecting hair's natural moisture, which means it won't dry you out. I've sent two bottles overnight, express mail.
—Maureen

MEDIUM   Kiehl's Protein Concentrate Shampoo for Oily Hair ($13.50)
www.kiehls.com

Shopping for the right hair care products isn't easy, and it gets particularly difficult for those with oily hair when just about every hair care line is primarily designed to add moisture or deep condition. Hair that gets greasy quickly is much more difficult to combat. The key is to wash hair daily, and the Kiehl's Protein Concentrate Shampoo for Oily Hair is a great product because the formulation has additional cleansing strength for oil-prone scalps.

LOW **Dove Beautifully Clean ($3.69)**

Mass retailers

You'll say good-bye to bad hair days with Dove Beautifully Clean. Dove thoroughly cleans hair without stripping, and can be used daily. Alternate with Dove Beautifully Clean 2 in 1 Shampoo and Conditioner with weightless moisturizing.

THE AUTHORS' PICK is the Phytopanama, though we loved the Dove Beautifully Clean almost as much. The Phytopanama just edges out the Dove when you compare cost with results.

HAIRCUT TIMING TIPS FROM DOVE CELEBRITY STYLIST EVA SCRIVO:

"Long hair should be trimmed about every two months to maintain health and shape. Shorter hair requires slightly more upkeep to maintain the style, so visit the salon every six weeks. For highlights, see your stylist every six to eight weeks. When possible, schedule haircut and highlighting appointments on the same day so the stylist can place your highlights in a pattern that is most flattering to your cut."

Fine/Thin Hair Shampoos

Does your scalp show more skin than a *Penthouse* Pet? Are you starting to envy the curly locks of Patrick Stewart? While thin may be in everywhere else on your body, it's not up top. There are products you can use to help fill in the blanks.

MEDIUM **Nioxin Bionutrient Protective Cleanser ($12.99)**

Fine salons or www.nioxin.com

This is the hands-down favorite shampoo of anyone with fine/thin hair. While Nioxin has certainly been around awhile, it has remained a well-kept secret . . . until now. It is important to note that the Bionutrient Protective line is for chemically treated hair and the Bionutrient Active line is for nonchemically treated hair. In fact, Nioxin has so many product lines that it can be more than a little confusing, which is why we're here to help you through the conundrum!

MEDIUM **bc bonacure Volume Shampoo from Schwarzkopf Professional ($12.50)**

Fine salons or (800) 707-9997

Bad hair can cause the type of day-to-day stress that brings sleepless nights, days of torment covering your head with hats, or even a rush trip to the nearest salon for a quickie cut that becomes a shortcut to disaster. We love this conditioner because it actually targets the dry areas of your hair to make it stronger and repairs damage only where needed.

LOW **L'Oreal VIVE Non-Stop Volume Root-Lifting Shampoo ($3.59)**

Mass retailers

Although poor nutrition, genetics, or hormonal changes may have gotten you to this place of thinning hair, don't worry. A body-building and root-lifting shampoo like this one will invigorate the scalp to speed up blood flow and supply more nutrients to your roots. If your hair is fine, blow-dry your hair in the opposite direction you intend to style it. Once you flip it to the styling direction this encourages root lifting and adds body to your hair.

THE AUTHORS' PICK is the Nioxin for Paula since she has thinner hair and is most impressed by Nioxin's results. Although Maureen's hair is anything but thin, she prefers the bc bonacure in any category because it yields spectacular results across the board.

HAIR TIP: To get your hair to grow faster, stronger, and healthier, Dr. Jeffrey Epstein, a plastic surgeon and expert in hair restoration in New York City and Miami offers the following suggestions:

➤ Vigorously massage your scalp while shampooing. This stimulates the follicles, which encourages the hair to grow.

➤ Flip your head and brush dry hair from root to end. Do this every other day.

➤ Exercise. A pounding heart pumps more blood to your hair follicles.

➤ Try Nioxin hair care products for fine or thinning hair, including shampoo, conditioner, and several other products. While promoted for regrowing hair, they seem to volumize the hair by strengthening and thickening the cuticles, thus providing a fuller look. For hair that is dry and prone to breakage, try bc bonacure Repair. This shampoo strengthens the hair with its botanicals, while gently but thoroughly cleaning the scalp. They are available at many upscale hair salons.

➤ Use Head & Shoulders or Nizoral shampoo several times a week to help block the effect of testosterone at the scalp level, which may help slow down hair loss and promote hair growth.

➤ Take B vitamins, biotin, and zinc, which play a role in promoting healthy hair growth. They're commonly found in multivitamins designed for thinning hair.

➤ One aspirin a day is not only good for your heart, but in women has been shown to reduce the risk of stroke. For anyone with or at risk for hair loss, it may also promote hair growth.

➤ The T3 Tourmaline Comb ($5.50, fine salons, or www.t3tourmaline.com) is antistatic, helping to smooth the hair and reduce breakage. The teeth are rounded and hand-finished, not sharp and pointy. Tourmaline naturally emits negative ions, which smooth the hair's cuticle. When the cuticle is not smooth, hair scales catch on one another, leading them to tangle and tear.

➤ The T3 hair dryer, also manufactured by Tourmaline, is up to 60 percent faster than any hair dryer on the market because it emits infrared heat, which penetrates the hair more deeply and dries it faster. This not only saves time but also reduces the amount of stress on the hair ($200, fine salons nationwide, or www.t3tourmaline.com). See page 25 for more information on the T3 and other hair dryers.

Normal Hair Shampoos

When it comes to hair, normal is a miracle. Most of us are either way too dry or way too oily, so rejoice if your hair is normal. You can use a wider range of products, and unlike the rest of us, who go through hundreds of treatments just to end up with the same old problems, you normal-hair types have many fewer bad-hair days.

HIGH Bumble and Bumble Alojoba Shampoo ($24.99)
Fine salons or www.bumbleandbumble.com

The exotic scents of this moisture-rich hair smoothie transport you to the sandy shores of Fiji, where a bronzed French dive instructor named Pascale is not interested in the fact that you have a degree in biochemistry from M.I.T. He's interested in a completely different set of frontal lobes, and he's going to show you how they make Alojoba, mon! This shampoo makes your hair super soft and silky.

HIGH Philip B. African Shea Butter Shampoo ($22.50)
Fine salons or www.philipb.com

Philip B. African Shea Butter Shampoo is rich yet lightweight, moisturizing, fragrance-free, and color-safe. It is a gentle conditioning shampoo for all hair types. The mild pH of 5.5 and the penetrating hydrators help to retain color longer. Shea butter comes from a tree nut that has healing and natural sunscreen qualities. Philip B. African Shea Butter Shampoo is also enhanced by pure plant extracts along with vitamin B_5 to increase manageability, moisture, and shine without weighing down hair.

MEDIUM bc bonacure Repair Shampoo from Schwarzkopf Professional ($11.90)
Fine salons or (800) 707-9997

bc bonacure's revolutionary (pH-adjusted) ApHinity technology actively targets problem areas, strengthens hair, and selectively repairs damage only where needed. It includes botanicals such as natural honey extract, which strengthens hair structure, and nourishing wheat proteins to repair, smooth, and seal the hair's outer cuticle surface for a polished glow and protection against further damage.

LOW Alberto VO5 Shampoo for Normal Hair ($.99)
Mass retailers

Like an old friend, Alberto VO5 never disappoints. You can't overuse this shampoo, particularly if you have normal hair, and since it's infused with a plethora of vitamins your hair is sure to stay healthy.

THE AUTHORS' PICK is the bc bonacure Repair Shampoo. It always makes your hair look beautiful and clean without residue, and the price compared to the results puts it over the top. Also, our publisher loves it and you can't really argue with that.

Highly Textured, Curly, Coarse, Hard to Manage, Overly Stressed, Color-Treated, or Generally Ornery Hair Shampoos

Chemical processing, sun, wind, genetics, and poor handling can leave your hair brittle, rough, and weak. If your hair fits into this category, the best way to treat it is to moisturize as often as possible. Here are some great shampoos to help you replenish those moisture levels.

HIGH Ojon Ultra Hydrating Shampoo ($18)
www.ojonhaircare.com

Maureen:

The expedition has taken a detour. We are now on the Caribbean coast in the Mosquitia region of Central America. The men and women here are well known for their beautiful hair and I have uncovered the secret. They use a palm nut oil extracted from the native Ojon tree to keep their hair silky and healthy. I am unbelievably amazed with the results, even on my dry and chemically treated hair. I have already packed several vials to bring back. Keep this a secret until the book is ready.

—Paula

Ojon Ultra Hyrdrating Shampoo is rich and gentle, and the ideal shampoo for extremely dry or unruly hair. It is also completely safe for chemically treated hair of all types. It has been the elixir used by the Miskito Indians, also known as the Tawira or "people of beautiful hair."

MEDIUM bc bonacure Repair Shampoo from Schwarzkopf Professional ($11.90)

Fine salons or (800) 707-9997

If keeping up with the Joneses is your thing, then you'll want this shampoo. Ever wonder why Mrs. Jones, with four kids under the age of ten and two dogs, never looks harried? It's because her shampoo is specially formulated to target only the problem areas, strengthen hair, and normalize weak or overstyled and chemically abused hair. With her hair in order, Mrs. Jones can easily solve the rest of the day's dicier moments and keep a cool head.

MEDIUM ELLiN LAVAR OptiMoist Shampoo ($10)

www.ellinlavar.com

This moisturizing shampoo is designed to gently yet thoroughly cleanse the hair while imparting a balance of amino acids and proteins into the hair for strength and elasticity. Its high content of moisturizers and conditioners keep the hair shiny and tangle- and static free while giving each strand a youthful appearance. It's powerful enough to use only once a week; don't overuse or you'll cross the line from taming your hair to beating it flat and lifeless. You want to show your hair who's boss, not assault it. Be sure to alternate this product with one of the other three in this category. It sometimes takes teamwork to tame the beast.

LOW L'Oreal VIVE Smooth-Intense Shampoo for Women of Color ($3.69)

Mass retailers

This godsend of a shampoo is made with camelina seed oil, which has an unusually high

REFLECTIONS ON COLOR

Hair that is color-treated has always been a challenge. Kerastase has launched a light-reflecting treatment that reveals mirrorlike radiance in colored hair. The line, Reflection, takes an aggressive stand with colored hair by actually smoothing and evening out the hair fiber, laying the foundation for optimal reflection. The Reflection line includes Bain Miroir shampoo ($29), Chroma Reflect Radiance—Enhancing Masque ($58), and Chroma Protective Polishing Cream ($34), all available at your nearest fine salon, or call (877) 784-8357.

natural content of cholesterol to smooth the hair. For highly textured hair, or hair that is intensely damaged from the sun or overbleaching, the results are transforming.

THE AUTHORS' PICK is the Ojon Ultra Hydrating Shampoo. If your hair is more difficult than Chinese algebra, the Ojon is the multifunction calculator to solve it.

Clarifying Shampoos

A clarifying shampoo has one job: to remove buildup of shampoo, gel, mousse, pomades, and other products that weigh your hair down with regular use. It differs from a regular shampoo in that it has an elevated acid content, and thus, it should be used sparingly, depending on the level of buildup on your hair. Use clarifying shampoos weekly for heavy buildup, biweekly for moderate buildup, and monthly for minimal buildup (if you don't use much product on your hair).

"Over time, all products that you use regularly on your hair will begin to build up and not be quite as effective due to the weight they create on you hair's cuticle," says celebrity stylist Oscar Blandi. "Think of clarifying shampoos like the exfoliate you would use on your skin periodically. It's like hitting restart!"

HIGH Soda Shampoo by Fresh ($24)
www.fresh.com

Soda shampoo is formulated with bicarbonate of soda bubbles, which adds volume while simultaneously removing residue from product buildup. The stimulating mint and lavender waters revitalize the scalp and enhance body and shine, while the grapefruit gives it an exhilarating scent. This shampoo is ideal for all hair types and best used weekly for clarifying action.

MEDIUM Oscar Blandi Shampoo D'Alternanza ($20)
www.oscarblandi.com

D'Alternanza is a very gentle clarifying shampoo with chamomile and aloe vera that should be used no more than once a week to remove buildup without stripping hair. Follow with your regular conditioner.

MEDIUM frédéric Fekkai Apple Cider Clarifying Shampoo ($18.50)
www.sephora.com

Good for all hair types, this shampoo rids hair of product buildup, chlorine, and environmental impurities. Real apple cider vinegar clarifies the hair while apple, rosemary, verbena, and kukui nourish and protect it. It deep cleans but does not strip the hair of its essential oils.

LOW Neutrogena Anti-Residue Shampoo ($4.99)
Mass retailers or www.drugstore.com

Neutrogena Anti-Residue shampoo was one of the first in its category and still maintains its reputation at the top of the heap. Used weekly, it instantly removes up to 70 percent of dulling residue buildup caused by continuous use of shampoos, conditioners, and styling aids. It cleans hair gently, rinses thoroughly, and can be used on all hair types. Better yet, the mild formula won't cause irritation.

THE AUTHORS' PICK is a split decision. Paula loves the Oscar Blandi Shampoo D'Alternanza because she uses so many products to get her dry hair soft and silky that the buildup after about two weeks is unbearable. The D'Alternanza strips the hair clean and keeps it shiny and healthy. Maureen loves the Soda Shampoo by Fresh. It is extremely gentle for a clarifying shampoo and it is almost impossible to overuse it, a virtue since the purpose of a clarifying shampoo is to strip your hair. It is still recommended that you use it only once or twice per week.

Color-Depositing Shampoos

Like those banking computer programs that round off and add fractions of cents, color-depositing shampoos and conditioners add minute amounts of color to your highlights. However, like those programs, a few days of use can add up to some serious amounts, so you will not have to visit the colorist as frequently. Color-depositing shampoos can enhance your colors, natural and otherwise, and make subtle changes to your look.

HIGH frédéric Fekkai Baby Blonde Shampoo and Brilliant Brown Shampoo ($28.50)

Fine salons or www.sephora.com

The challenge here is that Mr. Fekkai has created only two shades for his color-depositing shampoos: blonde and brown. But they both work phenomenally well and contain loads of natural ingredients to brighten your color and add shine.

MEDIUM DevaBlonde Low-Poo, DevaRed Low-Poo, DevaBrown Low-Poo ($14)

www.devachansalon.com

NOTE: These products are not shampoo, and if we refer to them as shampoo the company will have our heads. They, in fact, want it completely clear that these are "cleansers" and not sham-

poos because they contain very low doses of sodium laureth sulfate (SLS)—the ingredient that gives shampoo lather and also strips your hair of its natural defenses—hence the moniker Low. They also make No-Poo, which contains no SLS but also has no lather, which can be a confusing hair washing experience if you're not used to cleansing your hair without the poo. Each shade has a clever name—Calling All Blondes, SacRed Love, and Chocolate Lust—and they should be used like every other shampoo to neutralize those unwanted yellows or brassy tones that can rear their ugly heads.

MEDIUM ARTec color-depositing shampoo ($12.50)

Fine salons or (866) 849-4095

This is the no-contest favorite of every stylist we polled. As Kyle White, celebrity stylist at the Oscar Blandi Salon in New York City, says, "ARTec deposits the correct amount of color and gives your hair the right amount of change without being too much. It also fades evenly and washes out nicely." ARTec comes in multiple shades.

THE AUTHORS' PICK is ARTec. Color-depositing products can be very inconsistent, but ARTEC truly provides the highest quality and consistently the truest color.

Conditioners

Conditioner is your shampoo's wingman—without it your hair is dangerously exposed to the attacks of sun, dirt, and temperature changes. Always keep your hair safe and protected with a proper conditioner.

Dry Hair Conditioners

Your personality may be dry, but your hair shouldn't be. Dry hair has insufficient moisture and oil content, that may result from excessive washing, harsh detergents, a dry or hostile environment, inadequate diet, or even underlying diseases. Unlike a dry flower garden, the solution to dry hair is not always just to add water. Arid, flyaway locks need lots of TLC, and that means the right products with moisture-rich ingredients.

HIGH Oscar Blandi Shampoo di Jasmine Smoothing Conditioner ($20)

www.sephora.com

The secret is the jasmine. The delicate and captivatingly sweet fragrance will have you hooked. Beyond the scent, the jasmine oil smooths the hair and preps it for prestyling frizz control. Aromatherapists believe jasmine can be useful as an antidepressant; as a calming agent to soothe stress, pain, and anxiety; and as an aphrodisiac. So if it doesn't cure your stressed hair, it may be more effective than a session with your therapist.

MEDIUM bc bonacure Moisture Conditioner from Schwarzkopf Professional ($14.50)

Fine salons or (800) 707-9997

With the right information, anything is possible. We've already told you that the bc bonacure line actively targets dry areas and selectively repairs damage only where needed. It's a clever and discriminating conditioner for dry, curly, or permed hair.

LOW Pantene Pro-V Daily Moisture Renewal Conditioner ($3.99)

Mass retailers

Pantene Pro-V Daily Moisture Renewal Conditioner deeply penetrates the hair and insulates each strand to seal in moisture and protect against damage. It adds just the right amount of moisturizers where needed. Hair stays healthy, shiny, and virtually split-end free.

THE AUTHORS' PICK goes to the bc bonacure Moisture Conditioner from Schwarzkopf Professional. We admit that the Pantene Pro-V is more readily available, but we've been completely seduced by the bonacure line and its effectiveness on the hair.

Oily Hair Conditioners

Oil can be a good thing with hair, but too much oil every day is a slippery slope. Oily heads produce more oil than normal, and this requires gentle cleansers and conditioners to keep the oil at bay.

HIGH Kiehl's Hair Conditioner and Grooming Aid Formula 133 ($26)

www.kiehls.com

Formula 133 is a free-flowing detangling and conditioning rinse. It can be used after shampooing or as a conditioning and grooming aid anytime. It's particularly effective with normal to oily hair.

MEDIUM Korres Camelia Milk Conditioner ($17.50)

Fine salons

Made in Greece, Korres Camelia Milk Conditioner is especially formulated for oily hair. It forms a protective film on the hair shaft to seal in moisture, protect, and smooth. It detangles hair without buildup and contains antioxidant rich camelia milk, plus aloe vera and vitamin B$_5$ for long-lasting hydration.

LOW Dove 2 in 1 Shampoo and Conditioner ($3.69)

Mass retailers

For any other hair type this would not be so genius, but oily heads will appreciate that a 2-in-1 product will not overcondition.

THE AUTHORS' PICK in this category goes to Dove 2 in 1 Shampoo. If you've ever been skeptical of a 2-in-1 in the past, this product will turn you around.

Normal Hair Conditioners

Those of us who are hair-challenged (oily heads or dry heads), are insanely jealous of those of you with normal hair. But don't start gloating yet, because normal hair needs everything dry and oily hair need, perhaps just a little less depending on the season.

HIGH Pomegranate Conditioning Hair Rinse by Fresh ($24.00)

www.fresh.com

Fresh Pomegranate Conditioning Hair Rinse is a weightless daily conditioner that's suitable for all hair types. It detangles and moisturizes while adding amazing body, texture, and sheen to the hair. Pomegranate extract, a naturally derived antioxidant, and sunflower extract safeguard hair from the sun and other harsh elements.

MEDIUM bc bonacure Repair Conditioner from Schwarzkopf Professional ($13.90)

Fine salons or (800) 707-9997

Schwarzkopf's revolutionary (pH-adjusted) Ap-Hinity technology actively targets problem areas, strengthens hair, and selectively repairs damage only where needed. It leaves hair soft and manageable, and smooths and seals the hair's outer cuticle surface for a polished glow and to protect against further damage.

LOW Finesse Conditioner, Enhancing for Normal Healthy Hair ($5.49)

Mass retailers

Every Finesse product contains an exclusive silk protein formula to smooth the hair and improve the cuticle so that each and every strand is soft and silky. It's gentle enough for everyday use and it softens and adds manageability while maintaining the natural balance of healthy hair.

THE AUTHORS' PICK is bc bonacure Repair Conditioner, which is hands-down the best conditioner for normal hair. It's an extremely high-quality product for a reasonable price.

Fine/Thin Hair Conditioners

It's true that you can never be too rich or too thin, except up top where being thin is definitely not in. Here's the skinny on fine or thin hair: the core of thinner hair is more narrow than normal hair, which means that the actual diameter of the hair is smaller. Fine hair is more susceptible to damage, it tangles more easily and it doesn't hold a hairstyle as well, which means you need to be selective with hair products. The good news is that we have discovered a few great products to help you sashay through the cocktail season with thick, luscious locks instead of limp ones.

MEDIUM Nioxin Bionutrient Protectives Cleanser ($12.99)

Fine salons

Nearly every expert on our panel and everyone we spoke to with fine/thinning hair voted this the best conditioner. Conditioners for this hair type are also pretty tricky because fine/thin hair can become weighed down if the formulation is not perfect. The company boasts a host of rare, protective herbs and botanicals to help safeguard the scalp from drying.

Note that the Nioxin Bionutrient Actives offers the same great benefits as the Protectives but the Actives is specially formulated for nonchemically treated hair.

LOW L'Oreal VIVE Non-Stop Volume Conditioner ($3.59)

Mass retailers

No more wrestling with fine, thin hair. Most women who have this hair type find that conditioners give a horrid effect of weighty lifelessness. This truly revolutionary shampoo and conditioner system adds weightless volume that lasts, guaranteed, up to eighteen hours. It's a silicone-free mix of styling polymers that props hair from the root without a heavy, thick coating.

THE AUTHORS' PICK is Nioxin. While it's more pricey than the L'Oreal, the results are immediate and amazing. Your hair simply feels thicker and stronger, and that's a real confidence builder when your hair is fine and/or thin.

Highly Textured, Curly, Coarse, Hard to Manage, Overly Stressed, Color-Treated, or Generally Ornery Hair Conditioners

You may like your men rough, but you want your hair smooth, and that's asking a lot from hair that's feisty. We've chosen products that will help emphasize your hair's versatility, texture, volume, body, and bounce. Listen up: poker-straight hair is over, ladies, so stop complaining and learn how to make your ferocious frock fabulous with these favorites.

HIGH Ojon Ultra Hydrating Conditioner ($18)

Fine salons or www.ojonhaircare.com

This is without a doubt the first truly hydrating shampoo and conditioner that works immediately and over time, with increasing benefits, and does not weigh hair down.

HIGH bc bonacure Total Repair Treatment from Schwarzkopf Professional ($19.50)

Fine salons or (800) 707-9997

This is the ultimate hair warrior of conditioners. Used weekly, it rebuilds structure in only five to ten minutes, creating soft, silky, and vibrant hair. It's a miraculous conditioner that is effective for all hair types.

MEDIUM ELLiN LAVAR SatinSoft Conditioner ($12)

www.ellinlavar.com

SatinSoft conditioner contains cupuaçu, the rain forest's answer to shea butter. Bottom line: it will tame your wildebeests faster than you can say "VIP sale at Barneys!"

LOW Alberto VO5 Hot Oil Treatment ($3.99)

Mass retailers

You might have seen this old-timer in your grandmother's medicine cabinet and chuckled to yourself, "There's Granny's Alberto VO5!" Well, guess what? It packs the same deep-conditioning punch today as it did back then. You will see the results in just one minute. The coolest thing about using the Alberto VO5 is that you still have to soak that tube of conditioner in a cup of boiling hot water for one minute. Your grandmother did it forty years ago, and you're doing it the same way today. Use weekly or more often if needed. (They also now make a shower-activated version that is just as effective.)

THE AUTHORS' PICK is Ojon Ultra Hydrating Conditioner. Continuous use brings soft, silky smooth hair without heavy residue, buildup, or hair resistance to the product. It just can't be beat.

Hair Masks and Deep Treatments

When your hair truly needs life support, give your head a spa vacation with one of the following outstanding hair masks. They'll moisturize, revitalize, repair, and replenish your hair.

OUTRAGEOUS Ojon Restorative Hair Treatment ($55)

Fine salons or beauty.com

This uniquely concentrated, versatile hair rejuvenator contains 100 percent Ojon palm nut oil to improve the condition of damaged, color-treated, or processed hair without weighing it down. Fortifying, rebuilding, and nourishing, it leaves hair extraordinarily shiny, silky, and manageable. Yes, it's expensive but thoroughly and completely worth the price. You'll get dozens of treatments from one package.

HIGH Phytocitrus Vital Radiance Mask ($32)

Fine salons

Phytocitrus prolongs and enhances the beauty of recently colored, highlighted, or permed hair. In

CALLING ALL BLONDES

There's an innovative new hair care and styling product line for blonde hair that is chemically treated, damaged, or lifeless in any way. Blonde-Aid (www.luxelab.com) makes it possible for you to keep those sun-kissed locks year round without the damage. The Blonde-Aid celebrity fan club includes Marcia Cross. (Yes, it works for redheads, too!)

addition, it smooths the cuticle layer to ensure maximum shine. Phytocitrus prevents your color from fading, promotes softness and bounce in permed hair, and adds exceptional shine.

HIGH Curlisto Deep Therapy Masque ($30)

www.curlisto.com

You've been planning the big vacation for months: the tickets are purchased, your ocean view is secure, and you've even upgraded your rental car from a standard to a luxury in anticipation of some much-needed time off. But while you're packing visions of the hot sun of the West Indies beating down on your already stressed-out locks, we urge you to reach for your Curlisto Deep Therapy Masque, which will keep your hair in tip-top shape.

MEDIUM Phytoplage After Sun Repair Mask ($22)

Fine salons

This reparative moisturizing mask contains rush nut oil, shea butter, keratin, and vitamin B_5—nutrition that's essential to hair that has been weakened by sun exposure.

LOW L'Oreal VIVE Smooth Intense Anti-Frizz Masque ($4.99)

Drugstores

Finding a good anti-frizz masque for dry, frizzy hair is no longer a stretch. L'Oreal blessed our tresses with this intensive hair masque that brings harmony back to your locks without sacrificing your wallet.

THE AUTHORS' PICK is the Ojon Restorative Hair Treatment. You can use it repeatedly and you will consistently get the same results, which is rare for any shampoo or conditioner in any category. This conditioner is—and we mean to go over the top here—a miracle. A wonder of modern science. A gift from above. Truly unique.

Leave-in Conditioners, Creams, and Balms

Leave-in conditioners, creams, and balms can be true hair lifesavers. They protect your hair against the elements, harsh blow-drying, curling, straight-irons, and anything that takes a toll on or stresses your tresses.

HIGH Bumble and Bumble leave in (rinse out) Conditioner ($18)

Fine salons or www.bumbleandbumble.com

DEEP-CONDITIONING TIP

For African American and textured hair types, apply a fortifying oil such as ELLiN LAVAR Textures Nourish Oil as a deep conditioner (it can be used on the body as well). Apply liberally to dry hair from scalp to ends and leave in for 15 to 20 minutes, then shampoo out. To increase penetration, cover with a shower cap or aluminum foil, which will retain heat for deeper conditioning. A time-saving option is to apply a smaller amount of oil directly after shampooing (dime- to quarter-size, depending on hair length and texture) and leave it in.

Great hair is a challenge no matter what your hair type, but it's much easier to achieve great results when you have a product that can be used two ways. This conditioner can be used either way; you can rinse it out before you step out of the shower or leave it in for extra moisturizing when you're still feeling the need for that little something extra to kick it up.

LOW Infusium 23 Leave-in Treatments ($5)

Mass retailers

It's a conundrum when you put this leave-in treatment in your hand. It's so thin and watery that you can't imagine it works, but we truly believe it's one of the beauty industry's top ten miracle products. Infusium 23 Leave-in Treatments include special ones for frizz control, for moisturizing, and for color-treated or permed hair. Each strengthens and repairs damaged hair and improves the texture and manageability of your strands.

THE AUTHORS' PICK is the Infusium for two good reasons: it's really cheap and works phenomenally well.

Infusium Hair Repair Tips for Fall and Winter

Women tend to experience some common hair and scalp problems during the chilly and frigid months. David H. Kingsley, Ph.D., a trichologist with British Science Corporation, hears many complaints about dry, brittle hair, limp hair, hair static, flaky scalp, and hair loss, to name a few. For these scalp conditions, Dr. Kingsley offers the following basic advice:

➤ **Dry hair** is often caused by colder temperatures outside and dry electric or gas heat produced inside the home and office. The extreme changes in temperature can cause a dramatic reduction in hair moisture, which results in hair becoming exceptionally dry, brittle, and more susceptible to breakage.

➤ **Limp hair** is mainly caused by lack of humidity in the air. During the summer months, naturally curly hair absorbs moisture, from the air and hair becomes wavy with more body. In the fall and winter, hu-

HOW TO USE DEEP CONDITIONERS

As a Deep-Conditioning Treatment: warm ½ teaspoon of product in the palms of your hands (more for longer hair) and distribute onto dry hair from scalp to ends. Leave on for ten to twenty minutes, then shampoo well.

As a Leave-In Conditioner: warm a small amount in the palms of your hands until it becomes a lightweight oil, and distribute thoroughly through towel-dried hair. Style as usual.

As a Shine Enhancer: heat a very small amount in the palms of your hands and smooth over the surface of dry-styled hair.

midity levels drop, meaning less moisture is available to infuse hair with extra body.

Solution: To battle the damaging effects of the winter weather, and help prevent dry, limp, broken hair, Dr. Kingsley suggests using products specifically designed to restore moisture to the hair, such as Infusium 23 Moisturizing Shampoo and Conditioner, which leaves hair with a soft and silky feel. It is also important to use a deep conditioner, such as Infusium 23 Power Pac, that helps to retain moisture and provides a barrier against further breakage.

➤ **Static** is also a problem for dry winter hair. Spurred on by brushing or combing, cold air triggers hair strands to become more electrically charged. Hair fibers repel one another creating flyaways, making hair more difficult to control.

Solution: To trap much-needed moisture in the hair during the winter months, Dr. Kingsley suggests using a deep conditioner, such as Infusium 23 Moisturizing Leave-in Treatment, and an antifrizz product, such as Infusium 23 Complete Frizz Control Treatment. Both these applications will not only heighten shine and manageability, they will also reduce static and tame frizz and flyaways.

➤ **Flaky scalp** is a very common problem that can be caused by a change in weather. During the fall and winter months, humidity decreases, thus causing the scalp to lose moisture. This loss of moisture can lead to an increase in flaking and irritation. Surprisingly enough, people with an oily scalp are more likely to have this problem because they tend to have more oil glands,

which makes the skin more vulnerable to moisture loss.

Solution: Deep scalp moisturizing treatments will help get rid this pesky problem. The trick is to understand the difference between dandruff and dry skin. If you are not prone to dandruff throughout the rest of the year, then chances are the temperature change has had a detrimental effect on your scalp. Whether it's a drugstore brand or a spa treatment, scalp therapy products will help moisturize and heal uncomfortably dry skin. A humidifier can also help reduce the problem.

➤ **Fall hair loss**, also known as "seasonal hair loss," is thought by many to be as normal as leaves falling from trees and is caused by extreme changes in temperature. If this happens to you every year, then most likely it is normal for you. However, you may want be checked out by a hair loss specialist to make sure there isn't some other problem.

Solution: While there may be no way to halt the actual loss, there are some tricks to minimize the thinner appearance, which can be embarrassing or even devastating. Using a hair care regimen designed specifically for fine hair, such as Infusium 23 Maximum Body Shampoo and Conditioner, will increase hair's natural body and leave it looking fuller.

Hair Time Traps

Celebrity stylist Mark Garrison shares the following suggestions for at-home care in a hurry:

➤ Wash hair every other day—it's actually better for the hair.

➤ For quick dries, don't overuse heavy conditioners, because they retain moisture, which prolongs the drying process.

➤ Wrap hair in a towel and squeeze out the excess before blowing dry.

➤ If you use hair spray, select an aerosol or dry version, because pump sprays contain more moisture and require more drying time.

➤ If your daily hair maintenance exceeds twenty minutes, you may want to consider a more time-sensitive style.

A Word on Hair Tools

Celebrity stylist Eva Scrivo recommends the following tools to keep hair healthy and looking its best:

➤ A boar bristle brush will give you greater control while styling your hair. Using natural bristles instead of nylon or plastic creates more tension on each section, which will help you achieve smooth, shiny hair.

➤ A wide-tooth comb will untangle wet hair, which is at its most fragile. Start by combing out the snarls at the bottom section of hair first, and work your way up.

➤ When purchasing a hair dryer, look for one that comes with attachments, such as an air-concentrating nozzle and a diffuser. Air-concentrating nozzles are great for straightening hair and eliminating flyaways. Diffusers can kick curls up a notch. If your dryer did not come with these attachments, it is possible to purchase them separately. Just bring your dryer to the store with you to see that the attachments fit.

➤ Curling irons and Velcro rollers can provide soft curls or waves and help to create more volume. To make curls look more natural and maximize length, wrap hair 3 or 4 inches from the root, leaving 1 or 2 inches of ends out of the iron or roller.

➤ A flatiron will help you achieve straight and sleek hair in a hurry. Quickly blow-dry your hair with the aid of a large, natural-bristle paddle brush. Then, use the flatiron to straighten hair, section by section.

Curl Enhancers

If you're longing for curls but you're afraid of a "curltastrophe," fear no more. A little flounce around the shoulders while you walk is the latest hair trend, and you know it's right when those soft, sexy waves have others turning heads and asking, "Is that your natural curl?"

DEVACURL QUICK TIP

"More than 65 percent of the population has naturally curly or wavy hair," says Lorraine Massey, author of the book *Curly Girl* and partner in the Devachan Salon in New York City. "To reach new curly heights, resist the temptation to use a blow-dryer, and let your hair dry naturally. Never touch your hair while it's drying, and only loosen curls from the end—never touch hair from the root, because this is where curls are most vulnerable."

Keep them guessing, but don't forget these curl call necessities:

HIGH   Oscar Blandi Curl Acception ($18)

www.sephora.com

It's nothing less than a hair conundrum when you can't get the curl you want, or you get the curl but can't shake the frizz. Oscar Blandi Curl Acception is a potential suitor when you need the right curl at the right time. Whether you're styling for a casual brunch or a night at the opera, this curl operator will make you look like a million bucks.

MEDIUM   OSiS Twist ($12.50)

Fine salons or (800) 707-9997

Whoever said silence was golden was dead wrong—at least when it comes to hair, that is. With OSiS Twist you can get the most amazing, soft curls in a flash. Even if you're passed over for that promotion for work, your hair will speak volumes.

MEDIUM   Philosophy Curly Head ($11)

Fine salons

If your hair is curly, you want it straight. If your hair is straight, you want it curly! Curly Head hair serum gives you the option—it can be used to help bounce a curl or diffuse a frizz. Either way, Curly Head gives you high-class hair that anyone could love.

LOW   Finesse Touchables Mousse, Curl Defining for Curly or Wavy Hair ($3.79)

Mass retailers

Finesse Touchables controls frizz for beautifully defined curls, and it's alcohol-free so it won't dry your hair. It's never too stiff or sticky and provides lasting volume and control.

THE AUTHORS' PICK is the OSiS Twist. It always works, no matter how much buildup is on your hair, and it also works fast, so you can get on with your day without worrying about your curls. It also works on all hair types, which is not always the case with curl-enhancing products.

Curl Queen Ouidad Answers Some Tough Summer Curl Questions

Ouidad, who is recognized far and wide as the curl expert, has been solving curly hair dilemmas for more than twenty-five years. When the weather heats up, curls need some calming. Exclusively for *The Beauty Buyble*, she gives some quick and thorough advice on some most frustrating curl conundrums.

➤ The key to keeping curls looking good in humid air is to make sure the cuticle of the hair is already "filled" with moisture and proteins before you step out the door. Doing so makes the cuticle unable to soak in

FOR YOUR CURLY-HEADED ANGEL

Curly kids will cry no more! Christo, the mastermind behind Curlisto Systems, recently launched the first hair care system for curly kids. The line features Tearless Shampoo ($12), Detangle Rinse ($12), Leave-in Conditioner ($15), and Spray Mousse ($18). www.curlisto.com

any additional moisture from the air, which can cause frizz. Ouidad Climate Control Gel ($17) is an essential styling aid during these months to fill that cuticle and add internal weight to the hair shaft by delivering essential amino acids and proteins to the hair.

➤ Sexy, beachy, wind-blown hair is simple to get if you know the proper techniques. Simply wash and condition locks, but leave the conditioner in the hair—don't rinse it out. Try Ouidad PlayCurl Volumizing Conditioner ($12) for added volume. Finger-comb curls back away from the hairline, and then use a wide scarf at the front hairline to hold hair away from the face, letting hair air-dry. This will create big, fun, tousled hair. When you're ready to wash the look out, the left-in conditioner will have penetrated any knots and keep tangles from occurring.

➤ Summer ponytails can also show off fabulous curls. Try this half-bun version: Secure hair into a low ponytail and then pull the bulk of the tail (mainly the top part) back up through the elastic, stopping halfway. This creates a knot base, but allows for curls to spill over the top for a trendier look. Leave a little length but still vary from the traditional ponytail by making a loop instead. Make a dramatic side part and slick hair back using Ouidad Clear Control Pomade ($25) and secure hair at the nape. Gently twist the ponytail into a loop and pull the tail end back through the elastic. This is a great romantic look.

Smoothing Aids /Antifrizz Serums

Does your hair look like a fright wig? Would the engineers at the Brillo Company be interested in your hair texture? Does your hair have more fuzz than an AM radio in the Lincoln Tunnel? Then you could use a smoothing aid or antifrizz serum to add gloss, shine, and smooth texture.

HIGH Phytodefrisant Botanical Hair Relaxing Balm ($22)
Fine salons or (800) 557-4986

"My best friend from college and I just met recently for the first time in fifteen years. I couldn't help looking at her hair, which had always been so dry and frayed. She told me her secret was Phytodefrisant Relaxing Balm, and I went out to get some immediately. She was right, it worked wonders, and I've now agreed to attend the class reunion—thanks to her!"
  —Genevieve Johnson, Michigan

MEDIUM ELLiN LAVAR LiquidGlass Smoothing Serum ($15)
www.ellinlavar.com

It promises more proteins and vitamin A than any soothing balm on the market, and whether you believe it or not, LiquidGlass softens hair and leaves it smooth and shiny, so you won't complain.

MEDIUM OSiS Magic Anti-Frizz Gloss Serum ($13)
Fine salons or (800) 707-9997

If a cup of coffee first thing in the morning gives you an instant buffer against the rest of the world, then OSiS Magic is the next most important barrier for the long haul. This lightweight antifrizz gloss serum magically finishes styles by controlling frizz, static, and flyaways without weighing down hair. Sunflower seed oil smooths the hair and adds shine and bounce to even the coarsest hair. For straight hair, apply while hair is wet and smooth while blow-drying. For a polished style, you can work it through dry hair with fingertips or comb.

LOW **John Frieda Frizz-Ease Lite Formula Hair Serum ($9.39)**
Mass retailers

If you want to up your shoe budget without getting a new job, you can cut back on your hair care spending with John Frieda Frizz-Ease. It transforms dry, frizzy-prone permed or color-treated

DAMN STRAIGHT!

New York City stylist Mark Garrison offers the following tips on getting hair flat-out fabulous:

➤ While hair is damp, work a straightening gel, such as Philip B's Drop Dead Straight Hair Straightening Baume, through the length of the hair, making sure to coat the ends. This will keep hair frizz-free.

➤ For extra-coarse hair, add a couple of drops of oil, such as Philip B. Rejuvenating Oil, to the straightening gel, and then work it through the hair. Use a blow-dryer and a round brush: start at the back of the head, taking small sections of hair (the amount the brush can hold firmly) and stretching the hair taut. Direct the dryer nozzle downward onto the hair shaft and move the brush down the length of the hair, through the ends. Repeat with different sections of hair until it is completely dry. Use clips to keep wet hair out of the way as you work. Make sure there is no moisture left in the hair or it will result in frizziness or bends in the hair.

➤ If you are going to use a flatiron, hair must be completely dry. Use the flatiron to create that drop-dead straight look that Jennifer Aniston, Madonna, and Gwyneth Paltrow love to flaunt. Note: Do not put any finishing product on the hair before you use the flatiron, or it can cause the hair to fry. Taking small, thin sections (no wider than the flatiron), slide the flatiron down the hair shaft, and make sure to keep it moving. Finish with a light pomade (silicone-based or oil-based) to add sheen and keep hair smooth as silk.

➤ Women with chemically relaxed hair should not dry their hair with a hair dryer. Rather, they should let hair dry naturally to keep hair in its best condition.

➤ Unplug the iron on rainy, hot, or humid days, because they're not the ideal scenario for the super-straight look. Instead, work with hair's natural tendencies, and put a clip on it. Hair accessories are a great way to create a fresh, new look.

hair into instantly smoothed locks. It unsnarls tangles and banishes split ends with state-of-the-art, microrefined silicones. Hair has brilliant shine without being greasy or stingy.

THE AUTHORS' PICK is OSiS Magic Anti-Frizz Gloss Serum. Glosses can be tricky; too much and your hair is greasy, too little and you end up reapplying, which invariably leads to too much. We found that with the OSiS, you can't really apply too much; it never feels greasy. Since this product has the lowest risk factor, it's our pick.

Straightening Aids

Your friends warned you about that perm, but you didn't listen. You wanted to have fun. Now they're calling you Q-tip. Stop the madness with a straightening aid. Come back to those beautiful wavy locks. All is forgiven, though thanks to the pictures from your company picnic, perhaps not forgotten . . .

HIGH Redken Straight, Hair Straightening Balm ($13.99)
Mass retailers

This is your emergency roadside assistance for hair! Excellent for naturally curly, frizzy, or permed hair, it temporarily straightens hair, protects against humidity, adds silky shine, and protects from heat.

LOW Dove Straight & Soft Sleek Styling Cream ($3.99)
Mass retailers

If a pumped-up atmosphere is what you crave, then this might not be the styling cream for you. Dove Straight & Sleek will smooth your hair and probably your nerves once you see how well it works.

LOW Pantene Pro-V Get It Straight Gel ($3.99)
Mass retailers

Pantene Get It Straight provides all-day straightening for reduced frizz and flyaways. It's a non-sticky formula that provides a smooth, sleek, luminous appearance.

THE AUTHORS' PICK is Pantene Pro-V, the best smoothing gel by far! It is no-nonsense straightening at a regular bargain.

IT'S ABOUT TIME

To get your hair super-straight, it takes about two hours before going out the door. Humidity begins to take its toll right away, so be sure to apply a sealant (wax, pomade, or silicone spray) for more lasting results.

Weather Warriors/ Styling Aids

Okay, so here's the deal with hair gels, creams, mousse, and so on: there are just too damn many of them. Instead of rating these products ad nauseum, we decided to tell you what they do because it's just all too confusing, don't you think? You can call us lazy, but keep your etiquette intact and don't say it to our faces.

POMADE combats dry, frizzy, fluffy hair by providing weight and is great for all hair types. Pomade should be applied to dry hair; stiffer formulas are best for fine hair and creamier formulas for coarse hair.

GEL repels moisture and is ideal for slicking hair back and for curly hair. Apply gel to wet hair—mix with a styling cream or pomade to soften the texture and avoid the hard hold.

SILICONE SPRAY repels moisture and provides a shield and shine for all hair types. Apply silicone spray on dry hair and avoid applying to roots on fine, thin hair. Comb silicone spray through curly hair before styling and reapply after hair is dry.

MOUSSE holds moisture for curly styles and helps set straight hair. Apply on wet hair.

HAIR CREAM holds moisture and is ideal for creating a textured look of separated pieces. Cream typically doubles as a styling product and leave-in conditioner. Use sparingly, applying first to ends of hair and working up the hair unless hair is very dry and thick.

SHINE ENHANCER makes hair silky and smooth and can be applied wet, before hair drying or wiped gently across dry hair to smooth and reflect light like silk.

Did You Know?

Creating beautiful styles is not the only reason to use styling products. Creams, sprays, and gels actually protect your hair strands by creating a barrier from heat damage from styling tools. Sure, they build up over time, and you'll want to use a clarifying shampoo to strip your strands and start fresh, but these products do amazing things for the hair. So don't be shy about using products; dig in and try them to find the ones that work best for you, and you'll also be protecting your hair!

RED CARPET LOOKS

Have you been glued to the television, watching all your favorite celebrities strut their stuff on the red carpet? Do you wish you could create their fabulous hairstyles on your own? Pantene celebrity stylist Brett Freedman, who tends to the tendrils of such A-listers as Gwyneth Paltrow, Kate Hudson, and Kirsten Dunst, has the secrets to creating all the red-carpet looks so you can show your own Oscar-worthy hairstyles.

QUICK TIP: For a textured beachy look without a head full of product, mix 2 to 3 tablespoons of sea salt crystals with 1 cup of water in a small spray bottle. Spray on damp hair if straight or wet hair if curly to get that textured look.

Loose and Layered

For longer, layered tresses, create a piecey, textured look with lots of natural waves, as seen on Joss Stone. First, apply an egg-size amount of Pantene Pro-V In Control Shaping Mousse to damp hair and blow-dry upside down, while scrunching fingers through hair to bring out the natural wave. Once hair is dry, apply a small amount of Pantene Pro-V Texture & Shine Defining Pomade to a few sections of the hair from root to tip for added separation and shine. Finish with a spritz of flexible hold hairspray to keep the style in place.

Super-Sleek Ponytail

To create a sleek, polished pony, apply Pantene Pro-V Smooth & Shine Styling Milk to damp hair before blow-drying straight with a paddle brush. This hybrid styler contains both conditioning agents and styling polymers that work to smooth out unruly, frizz-prone hair and provide long-lasting hold with shine. Then pull back the hair into a ponytail and secure at the nape of the neck. Add a little more product to the ends of the hair and go over with the blow-dryer one more time for an ultra-smooth finish.

Feminine Curls

Create flirty, feminine, retro-looking curls à la Marilyn Monroe. To get the look, use Pantene Pro-V Extra Fullness Gel to pump up thin hair for a thicker, fuller look. The formula contains thickening polymers that provide increased, long-lasting control for more defined styles. To create a full head of retro curls, work a quarter-size amount of gel through damp hair from root to tip. Blow-dry with a round brush and then secure hair in 2-inch sections with hot rollers and let sit for about twenty minutes. Once you remove the rollers, the gel will help keep the curls in place.

IONICALLY YOURS

When it comes to ionic hair dryers, the T3 is Orlando Pita's pick. "I love the T3 hair dryer because it's so different from any I've tried before. It's light, it's quiet, and when I started using it I realized the drying was going faster because it releases more heat. The hair had beautiful shine and silkiness to it, and there was no static electricity. You do need to move with it—you can't leave it in one place for too long. Be careful with it because it dries fast, which is better for your hair because it's exposed to heat for less time." Orlando has used the T3 on Jennifer Connolly, Anne Hathaway, and Gwyneth Paltrow.

Hair Dryers

Your husband/fiancé/boyfriend/cute guy down the block makes a huge freakin' deal over "having the right tool for the right job." Men tend to have enough tools in the garage to service the space shuttle, yet they use the same combination of hammer/screwdriver/duct tape/yellow pages to fix (or not) anything. You need top-of-the-line tools too, though you will actually be using yours.

Invest in a good hair dryer; it is the key tool to care for your third most visible asset (after the twins and the caboose). You'll spend a little more cash, but you'll really see the results in your hair. And what's another few bucks for something you'll use every day compared to that flanged drop-forged solid steel whatsit that he just had to have but has been using as a paperweight for that stack of old *Playboy* magazines in the basement?

Non-Ionic Hair Dryers

Non-ionic hair dryers are dryers that do not produce ionic conditioning. While ionic hair dryers produce millions of negative ions, which help to eliminate frizz and flyaways, many are also engineered to dry the hair faster and with higher levels of heat. If over-used, the results can lead to dry hair with more breakage and split ends. For these reasons, some people prefer to stick to the non-ionic hair dryer or alternate with an ionic hair dryer for optimal benefits.

HIGH Elchim 2001 Professional (Starting at $100)

Fine salons or (800) 875-7511

Orlando Pita, celebrity stylist to many famous heads in Hollywood, likes the Elchim Professional hair dryer. "You can buy it at any beauty supply outlet, and I like it because it gives strong heat. I need to work fast with my fashion shows, and heat is everything when it comes to time. The hair dryer I use has to work at the speed I need to get the models on the runway."

Professional stylists love the Elchim because it's lightweight and has more blowing options than Monica Lewinsky; switch combinations for seven ranges of speed and temperature.

MEDIUM Conair 1875 ($27.99)

Drugstores

This is a very groovy dryer because it comes in a super cool shade of blue, and it's translucent, so if you've ever wondered what's inside your dryer you can actually see the guts with this one. We also love Conair products because you can get them at any drugstore and they're reliable.

STYLING PRODUCTS FOR FLATIRONS

Ironing can fade hair color, but if you use good shampoos and conditioners you can prevent the fading. Use a shampoo and conditioning line that is designed for sealing in color, such as L'Oreal Kerastase Reflection line or Color VIVE by L'Oreal.

LOW Conair Euro Styler Champion ($19.95)
Drugstores

At $19.95 this dryer really packs a punch: it delivers 1900 watts of power and it's ultraquiet, which is unique for a hair dryer with this amount of power. The turbo power also means that it shortens the drying time so you can be party-perfect in seconds flat.

Ionic Hair Dryers

While most blow-dryers rely on heat and high-speed wind to dry hair, ionic blow dryers send negative ions to break up the water molecules faster, thus cutting drying time, often by half.

HIGH The Tourmaline T3 ($200)
Fine salons, (888) HairArt (424-7278), and www.t3tourmaline.com

The T3 uses tourmaline, a semiprecious gemstone that produces negative ions, which when combined with infrared heat, dries the hair from the inside out. The result: your hair will dry more than twice as fast as with traditional driers. Hair is also exposed to high heat for less time, eliminating frizz and damage. Celebrities who love it include Jennifer Lopez, Tyra Banks, Ashlee Simpson, and Paris Hilton.

HIGH Bio Ionic Hair Dryer ($165)
Fine salons or (888) 755-6834

This dryer makes even the most natural styles look sultry. The ion complex breaks down water faster, which transulates to super-fast drying time. The dryer also claims to preserve 58 percent more moisture to your hair. Although we can't prove the moisture factor, we can tell you that this is simply an amazing hair dryer and you will be impressed with ultrasmooth, silky hair. Oh, and it's extremely lightweight and quiet, too!

HIGH CHI PRO ($250)
www.farouk.com

This is a super-fast drying machine built for pure power and performance. Don't leave home without it!

LOW Conair Ion Shine 1875 Watt Hair Dryer ($18)
www.drugstore.com

In addition to the great price, easy availability, lightning speed, and pin-drop quiet performance, what you'll really love is the extra-long cord that comes with the Conair Ion Shine. What can we say? We can't resist anything with a long cable. This is the next best thing to a cordless, and you don't have to sacrifice drying power.

HEAT PROTECTION

When using a flatiron, always apply product beforehand to protect hair from heat. The unique Weightless Moisturizers found in Dove Straight & Soft Sleek Styling Cream ($4, mass retailers) provides a great barrier to help prevent hair damage from heat styling.

Flatiron

You've heard the stories of how, back in the day, your mother would flatten her hair with a clothes iron over the ironing board. When the ceramic tourmaline flatiron hit the market, it quickly replaced the automobile, the radio and yes, even the television as the twentieth-century's greatest invention. The heavens re-sounded with trumpets. God smiled. Angels wept. Woman had fire, the wheel, and now an easy and comfortable means of straightening her hair. Naturally, the "grass is always greener" sentiment applies here: if you have straight hair you want it curly, and if you have curly hair you want it straight. So, for those curly heads, here's some straight-up advice on the best flatiron.

HIGH T3 Flat Iron and T3 Wet-to-Dry Iron ($200)

Fine salons, (877) Sephora or www.sephora.com

The T3 Wet-to-Dry flatiron is ceramic, which al-lows for the cuticle to remain very flat and smooth. The tourmaline crystals help to seal the cuticle, which is why the hair comes out so shiny and silky. "I can get the hair smooth and straight without having to do the blow-dryer first and then the iron. This is ultimately better for the hair, be-cause you don't have to apply two types of heat to it," says Orlando Pita.

HIGH GHD Ceramic Styling Iron ($195)

Fine salons or www.folica.com

If you have to neaten up fast, the GHD will get you straight and chic in no time. Industry insiders say this is the Holy Grail of straightening irons. The GHD features a built-in microcompressor that conducts heat fast and retains it more effectively. The result is instant long-lasting heat for quick styling and poker-straight hair.

HIGH Farouk CHI Ceramic Hairstyling Iron ($180)

www.farouk.com

We love our CHI and you will, too. It heats up in milliseconds, or so it seems, and the hair is never dry after use. The CHI also locks in moisture and we love the way the swivel cord lets us move and groove as we straighten our strands.

MEDIUM Conair Instant Heat Ceramic Straightener ($29.99)

Drugstores

With twenty-five variable temperatures, this straight-ener is sure to please everyone. It heats up in sixty seconds and glides across the hair for instant, silky results.

LOW BaByliss Mini Ceramic Hair Straightening Iron ($19.95)

Fine salons

While this is certainly not the easiest straightening iron to find on the market, it is certainly the best in this price range. The BaByliss heats up fast, and more important, it cools down just as quickly so you can adjust the temperatures without poten-tially burning your hair.

Hair Sprays

If the hair dryer is the brush in the sculpture that is your hair, colors are the paints, and hair spray is the varnish in creating your masterpiece. It is what will make your creation last for posterity, or at least the 4:30 meeting. Hair sprays are not multipurpose. You need different types of hold for different effects and various situations.

With hair spray, you can definitely have too much of a good thing. Think of it as a finishing flourish, not as construction material. Your hair is intended to be silky and stay in place, not be a big ball of cotton candy perched on your head.

According to Dove celebrity stylist Eva Scrivo, aerosol mist is finer and more suitable for thin, fine hair. Nonaerosol pumps dispense more product with a single spray, making them more effective on thick or curly hair.

Light-Hold Hair Spray

HIGH Bumble and Bumble Does It All Styling Spray ($21)
Fine salons or (888) 728-6353

This virtually critic proof hair spray provides hair relief to woman across the country. It holds your hair without bulk or risk of falling flat, and you can brush through it without losing a modicum of hold. It also provides nice protective barrier against irons or rollers.

MEDIUM Oscar Blandi No Gravity ($18)
Fine salons or www.oscarblandi.com

We love this product because it has so many uses. It can be used as a styling aid to add body, texture, and support the root area, and No Gravity can support your entire do. The secret ingredients actually thicken the width of each hair strand to give your hair more volume by forming a scaffolding effect around your hair to hold it in place ever so gently.

LOW L'Oreal Studio Line Finishing Spray ($4)
Drugstores

What we love about the L'Oreal is that it gives you a very light, natural hold if you go over your hair with it once, but if you continue to spray, the hold increases. It also dries incredibly fast and doesn't make hair feel dry.

Medium-Hold Hair Spray

HIGH Phytovolume Actif Maximizing Volume Spray ($24)
Fine salons

We love Phyto because it consistently delivers excellent results. Created for fine/limp hair, it is a gentle spray with a solid hold that works well on all hair types.

MEDIUM Phyto Pro Strong Finishing Spray ($18)
Fine salons

This spray is perfect for all hair lengths and the hold is natural without being overdone. The best part, though, is that it brushes out easily, unlike most hair sprays, and even provides UV protection.

LOW Dove Flexible Hold Hairspray with Natural Movement ($4.29)
Mass retailers

This hairspray not only smells great, but it delivers the same results as the more expensive hair sprays. It also doesn't leave that sticky, tacky residue and washes out easily.

Maximum-Hold Hair Spray

HIGH Aveda Brilliant Hair Spray ($25)
Mass retailers

Keeping your style in place is one thing, but to keep it there with a hair spray that adds shine like this one is a bonus. We love it.

MEDIUM Paul Mitchell Freeze and Shine Super Spray ($12)

Mass retailers

This is virtually the most natural, nonsticky, maximum hold hair spray we've tried. It smells great and holds your hair in place without looking cemented on.

LOW Aussie Instant Freeze Spray ($4.19)

Mass retailers

A little goes a long way—one quick spray and you're done, and your hair will stay there all day. If you have a challenging hair style or difficult to control hair, you will be amazed with the way this spray keeps it all together, even in very hot, humid weather.

TRESemmé European Tres Two Hair Spray ($2.50)

Drugstores or www.walgreens.com

Totally touchable maximum hold hair spray is hard to find, but TRESemmé is readily available. Our experts like it because the mist is so fine; the hold is heavy, yet movable. It's a professional product at a drugstore price.

Color Pitch

Whether you're a teenager who is getting highlights for the first time, a young woman in her twenties who wants a more professional look as she enters the workforce, a fifty-year-old who wants to cover up unwanted grays, or simply a thirty-five-year-old woman looking for a change, hair color is important to women of any age. In fact, 60 percent of women regularly color-treat their hair. No matter how old they are, a major concern for these women is maintaining the vibrancy and richness of their color between salon visits and at-home processes. Pantene has a line of products to ease their worries. **Pantene Pro-V Blonde Expressions, Brunette Expressions,** and **Red Expressions** leave hair looking richer longer without depositing color. The three collections include shampoos, conditioners, treatments, and stylers that protect against color damage.

At-Home Hair Color

At-home hair colors have a questionable reputation, not unlike the dorky-looking girl in school with the braces, coke-bottle glasses, and the love of drab wool plaids. But you never

EVA SCRIVO'S PRECISION APPLICATION TIP

Root-lifting hair sprays are a fairly new concoction. They need to be carefully applied for maximum styling benefit. Use Dove Precision Volume Lift & Hold Hair Spray by holding the spray nozzle 6 to 8 inches from the head. Spray in quick bursts for no more than a second at a time. Target the root of the hair sections only and let the product dry before reapplying.

know; this girl may show up at the prom look-ing like Cinderella—sparkling and perfect. Don't be the girl in the peach and brown poly-ester prom dress. At-home hair color has come a long way and can take you from the back of the school bus to prom queen in less than one hour. Here are some home coloring kit fairy godmothers.

Since at-home hair color is by its very na-ture inexpensive, we've given you our ex-perts' top picks in only the high and low categories.

HIGH Féria Multi-Faceted Shimmering Colour ($18)

www.walgreens.com

The Feria multi-faceted system delivers pure color in varying shades throughout each strand of hair so that your color is not monotone and flat. This means that darker hairs will have a darker tone, and lighter hairs will have a lighter tone so that you look like you have professional highlights without the professional price tag.

LOW Garnier 100% Color Permanent Intense Gel-Creme ($7.99)

www.walgreens.com

Garnier delivers beautiful, rich shades that last without premature fading. The gel is also very gentle to the hair and provides optimal condition-ing and shine.

LOW Clairol Nice 'n Easy Permanent Hair Color ($7.99)

www.walgreens.com

Clairol Nice 'n Easy has long had a reputation for providing the best coverage for gray hair and each box comes with the ColorSeal gloss to lock in color. The ColorSeal gloss can also be used for up to six weekly treatments.

LOW Clairol Nice 'n Easy Root Touch-Up Kit ($6.99)

Mass retailers

This is hands-down voted the best root touch-up kit by our panel of experts. It's very easy to use, but if you are a root touch-up virgin, you need to figure out exactly how long to keep the product in your hair by testing it. "The best way to test is to do less time at first to see how it takes to your hair and then the next time you can go longer," says Kyle White, celebrity colorist at the Oscar Blandi Salon in New York City.

Lorri Goddard-Clark's Quick Color Tips

Celebrity colorist Lorri Goddard-Clark, whose cadre of celebrity clients includes Drew Barry-more, the Olsen twins, Raquel Welch, Kate Capshaw, and Hilary Swank, recommends Clairol and L'Oreal at-home coloring kits. "These are the two easiest to find, and they yield the best results." For highlights, Lorri likes the Clairol Frost & Tip kits.

Hot Tip #1: The most critical thing that is not given to you in the box is a barrier cream, or cream for the hairline, nape, and tops of ears. This is very important, because a good barrier cream prevents staining from the darker hair colors, such as browns, blacks, and reds. "My favorite is Vaseline. No more ring-around-the-hairline." But what if you're already *oopsed* and you're staring at a stained hairline? "The number one easiest way to remove it is with two very accessible, yet seemingly unlikely items," says Lorri. "Get some cuticle remover and cigarette ashes." Yes, you read that correctly. Burn a cigarette and collect the ashes. Mix them together lightly on a washcloth (first dip in the cuticle remover, then dip into the ashes), then rub that quirky concoction around the hairline and it will remove the stain. Do this before you shampoo for the second time from a fresh hair coloring. "This is an amazing trick that works wonders," Lorri says.

Hot Tip #2: The Smudge! It's three or four weeks since your last coloring and now you have that #2 pencil vibe framing your face. To soften it without having to run to the colorist every three weeks, purchase L'Oreal Preference home coloring kit in two shades; one shade somewhat lighter than your shade and ever so slightly darker. Mix ½ of each shade and use only one of the 2-ounce developer bottles. Lightly smudge the mixed color around the edge of your hairline, the nape of the neck, and around the ears and immediately wash out. Don't let it sit there; you're just smudging it. "This should soften your base and take the edge off. It's super-subtle, but makes all the difference in the world," says Lorri.

Hot Tip #3: Another great way to touch up your roots with highlighting is to purchase the Clairol Frost & Tip and a soft bristle toothbrush. Once mixed, barely pull through hairline, slicing through with the soft bristle brush. Let sit 7 to 10 minutes and shampoo, and you'll be amazed.

Are You a Color Virgin?

If you're having first-time color anxiety, Edita Robertson, senior colorist at the Mark Garrison Salon in New York City, gives the latest color lingo that you'll need to know before you take the plunge.

SEMIPERMANENT hair colors contain a small percentage of peroxide and no ammonia and can only darken hair. The roots need to be maintained with touch-ups every four to six weeks, but this is the least damaging color process for hair.

DEMIPERMANENT means there's peroxide but no ammonia. Again, this can only darken hair, and the roots need to be touched up every four to six weeks. Demipermanent is excellent for gray coverage.

PERMANENT color contains both peroxide and ammonia. It can make hair darker or a few shades lighter and lasts until the hair grows out. The roots need to be touched up every four to six weeks. The coverage is great for gray hair.

BLEACHING oxidizes the melanin (color) in your hair to a colorless compound. Once you bleach your hair there's no going back because the color has been permanently removed. The only way is to let your hair grow to its natural shade. If you want to go platinum blonde, you use a permanent hair dye, which contains bleach or bleaching agents, to achieve this effect.

GLOSSING/GLAZING is semipermanent color placed on the hair for a short period of time to darken hair slightly or change tonality (like ash blonde to golden blonde). Some glossing is clear and used just for shine, and either way it needs to be applied every few weeks.

HIGHLIGHTING means bleaching or permanent color to lighten hair. Highlights add a brighter dimension to hair color. This can be done delicately for a very natural look or by painting the highlights on for a blonder hue. The roots need to be touched up every three months.

LOWLIGHTS are permanent or demipermanent hair color used to break up an overlightened head of hair. The color is applied on hair using foils and provides a nice contrast against your base color. With lowlights you need to touch up roots as needed, typically every three months, and the process is often used to blend grays.

FOILING involves placing very fine sections of hair onto rectangular sheets of foil and applying color or lightener. The foil is folded to keep the color in place and is the closest application to the hair root of all the highlighting techniques.

BALIAGE is a lightener in the form of powdered bleach that is hand-painted onto select pieces of hair to emphasize a style. The color will grow out, but roots are not really an issue since the baliage process doesn't go that close to the root.

CHUNKING means taking large sections of hair and lightening them randomly, for the boldest highlighted look. This can be achieved through foiling or baliage as well.

FLASHING THE BASE means that a clear hair lightener is used to fill in the roots when they've grown enough to make your look a bit uncomfortable. Flashing is used to better spotlight very blonde highlights and is left on only for a few minutes.

Still confused? More Hair Highlights with Kyle White

We asked celebrity stylist Kyle White of the Oscar Blandi Salon in New York City for more tips on colored-treated hair.

When is the right time to color your hair, and what is the Marilyn Monroe Factor?

The right time to color your hair is NOW; everyone should try coloring their hair! If you don't, it's like having the same hairstyle your whole life, and that's boring. You don't have to do anything extreme, but even just a semipermanent color can add shine and texture, and a couple of highlights can change your whole look. In fact, there are very few things that can transform someone in just a couple of hours the way color can, and that's why criminals on the run always dye their hair first. I think hair color is something to have fun with as well because it's easily changeable (within reason) and can really change your life. Think about it. Marilyn was just Norma Jean until she went blonde, and who was Lucy till she went red? You can find the real you through color. Don't wait a minute longer. Color your hair now.

How do I know what color is right? If I'm in a rock band, should I go blue?

When figuring out what hair color is right for you, lifestyle and maintenance should be taken into consideration. There are three main factors to look at, and the most important is skin tone. Warm skin tones (complexions with pink and red in them) should try to stick to cool tones (*blonde* and *light brown*), because they will play down the pink in your face. The ashy or olive skin tones (complexions with green tones in them) should stick with warmer tones (dark *brown* and *black*) for the same reason. They warm up their faces, making them less green. Neutral skin, such as Drew Barrymore's, can go both ways. Of course there's an exception to every rule. If you're in a rock band and want to dye your hair blue, does it really matter what your skin tone is?

The second consideration is eye color. Lighter eyes tend to look more natural (if that's what you're going for) with lighter hair colors, and darker eyes tend to look more natural with darker hair colors, but once again there are always exceptions. Black hair and blue eyes can be fabulous, but you have to have the right face. If you're thinking about doing something like that, you should consult a professional, because if it's not fabulous it's nothing short of horrible!

Finally, the time of year affects how your hair should look and how the world sees you. A few highlights in the summer when you are getting a little tan and the sunlight is more yellow can perk up your color and brighten everything, including your skin. Slightly deeper color in the winter adds warmth to your skin and keeps you from looking washed out.

What are the best color options for gray hair, and what if I'm commitment-phobic?

It depends on how much gray you have. If it's just a few strands here and there, then a semipermanent color is the way to go because it has a very low volume of peroxide (if any) and no ammonia. Semipermanents add texture and shine, but best of all they gradually wash out so there's no commitment. Plus, if something goes horribly wrong you know that in a few shampoos most of it should be gone. If you have more than 30 to 40 percent gray, then you need permanent color. Try to stay within a shade or two of your natural hair color, as these products have peroxide and can strip your natural color. If you go too light, that could mean a head full of orange. If you're naturally light brown to dark blonde and there are a few grays popping out you, could try camouflaging it with a few strategically placed highlights. All of these things can be done in the salon or with drugstore brands. I recommended the Garnier products because I believe they deliver the truest shades.

Why does my hair color fade?

Hair color fades for a variety of reasons. One of the biggies is oxidation, the chemical reaction that happens when oxygen attaches itself to color molecules. This causes fading and dulling. The sun is a big color fader as well, and that's why museums never hang art in direct sunlight. You may also have noticed that the sun kills the paint job on a new car over time. If you like your hair color, keep it covered in the sun and it will last much longer. The shampoo you use and water you have can also affect your color. Hard water or well water with mineral deposits can cause color to go drab, and harsh or medicated shampoos strip your hair and thus strip the color as well. If you bought a Porsche you would use the best high-octane, unleaded gasoline you could find, right? Well, your hair color is the same, so make sure you're using a quality shampoo made for color-treated hair, and possibly a color enhancer such as the ARTec product line. All of these help to prevent fading.

How do I know when it is necessary to do touch-ups? Why does Sarah Jessica Parker always show dark roots?

It depends on how fast your hair grows, how much gray you have, and how far you have strayed from your natural color. Someone with dark brown hair who has dyed her hair platinum will need to touch up every three to four weeks, while someone with dark brown hair who dyed it medium brown might need to touch up only every eight. I always tell people that you will just know—you don't have to be a hair colorist to look in the mirror and see that you have gray roots down to your ears and you need a touch-up. Some people (like Sarah Jessica Parker) actually like dark roots, which I think on the right girl can be cool, but gray roots are always bad. I say as a general rule that six to eight weeks is a good time to take a look in the mirror and see what's what, then make your own decision.

Is it dangerous to go too blonde?

One of the dangers of going too blonde is washing out your skin tone. You never want your hair the same color as your face, or you'll wind up looking like a corpse. The process of blonding hair requires removing pigment, which can be a harsh process, so going very blonde can really do a number on your hair. Overprocessed blonde hair can leave you with a head full of straw or something resembling a cotton swab. I think blonde is the most complex color to do because you can go from supermodel to topless dancer in two shades. Every once in a while step back and take a look at yourself and make sure your hair looks healthy and is not blending in with your face, and if no one has asked for a lap dance lately (other than your husband or boyfriend), then you're probably okay.

What type of shampoo is best for color-treated hair?

One that is pH balanced, with extra conditioners and low surfactant levels (so that it doesn't strip your color). I absolutely love Oscar Blandi Crema shampoo and conditioner for color-treated hair.

How often should I use a clarifying shampoo, and how do I treat my dandruff without it?

If you color your hair, avoid clarifying shampoos, which are made to remove product buildup and mineral deposits, pollutants, and so on from the hair. They will also remove color molecules, and shampoo with heavy detergents will fade color, as will any medicated shampoos that contain tar. People who have scalp conditions that require these types of shampoos should coat their hair with conditioner, use the medicated shampoos on their scalp (that's what needs the tar, not their hair), and then use a shampoo for color-treated hair after that.

How do I protect my hair color from the sun?

Use a sunscreen for the hair. I recommend Phytoplage and the Kerastase Red Line because these products are specifically designed to protect the hair from sun exposure. Each of these products contains sunscreens. If you think about it, even if you apply SPF 30+ sunscreen to your face and body, if you go to St. Bart's for a week you'll still get tan because the sun is so strong. The same goes for your hair, only it won't tan, it will just get terribly damaged. I always suggest floppy hats or a chic silk scarf when on the beach. A leave-in protein such as the Oscar Blandi Jasmine Protein Mist is great for strengthening and protecting the hair, and a conditioning mask once a week is also a good idea.

I have been cheating on my colorist. Am I now damaged goods?

Cheating on your hair colorist once in a while is okay because it gives you a new perspective on your hair color. Also, like Dorothy in *The Wizard of Oz*, you may find yourself saying, "There's no place like home." But if you do cheat, just keep something in mind: we always know!

PART 2

FACE

Let's face it, we spend a lot of time looking at other people's faces and our own. This is one area where you don't want to read between the lines. The right makeup and skin-care products can be the difference in having others call you "ma'am" or getting carded in the liquor store when you're well over twenty-one. Which would you prefer?

Face Moisturizers

Choosing the right moisturizer for your skin is right up there with finding the right man. Use the wrong moisturizer and your skin screams "get me out of here," just like you if you have the wrong man in your life. We asked New York dermatologist Dr. Doris Day some key questions about facial moisturizers, and here's what she had to say:

How should you select the right moisturizer for your face?

➤ You lose more water from your skin at night than you do during the day, so you should use a moisturizer that is richer at night. I see so many people who don't moisturize at night, and they use drying products for acne or antiaging treatments. They wake up with dry skin, so they use a rich moisturizer in the morning. Then they get breakouts and try to fix it with the drying product at night. What they need to do is moisturize at night, use a lighter moisturizer during the day, and always use SPF in their moisturizer during the day.

➤ Use products that are designed for the face. Those with SPF are good for the daytime.

➤ Oil-free does not mean "no oil," it means that the word oil is not in the ingredient list (it's very sneaky). If you want products that are less likely to clog pores, look for the words non-acnegenic or non-comedogenic.

➤ "Unscented" may have a masking scent, "scent-free" means there is no added scent.

What ingredients should you look for in a moisturizer for dry skin, oily skin, combination skin, stressed or irritated skin, young skin, or skin with acne?

➤ For acne-prone skin I like low concentrations of salicylic acid. I developed a line for Estée Lauder Company called good skin

---

MOISTURIZER QUICK TIP

"When using a moisturizer without sunscreen, first apply the sunscreen, then moisturizer," says Dr. Dennis Gross, a dermatologist in New York City. "Think of sunscreen like a coating that clings to the skin—it clings better when in contact with bare skin. Conversely, the presence of moisturizer obstructs and compromises the tight bond onto the skin by the sunscreen."

(www.goodskindermcare.com) that has an excellent line for acne prone skin. It contains antiaging ingredients, along with antiacne ingredients, since so many of my acne patients are also fighting off wrinkles. I also have in the line an excellent SPF 30 lotion for acne-prone skin.

➤ For skin that is typically irritated I recommend any facial moisturizer with shea butter, hyaluronic acid, and pentapeptides.

➤ For oily skin or skin with acne you want a good moisturizer with dimethicone, salicylic acid, tea tree oil, and vitamins A and C.

➤ For combination skin, look for ingredients that include botanicals; hyaluronic acid; vitamins A,C, and B; and pentapeptides.

What is your daily skin care regimen?

I wash twice daily with a milky cleanser. I use the good skin's Soft Skin Creamy Wash. Then I use the All Firm serum I made for good skin. After this I use my All Calm SPF 25 lotion. At night, after washing I use the serum, followed by Renova or Avage (prescription antiaging creams) with my All Calm Moisture cream over that. I exfoliate with my All Bright Two-Step Peel pads twice per week (step one contains citric acid along with lime extract, and step two

has sodium bicarbonate to neutralize the peel and aloe and hyaluronic acid to soothe and hydrate the skin). In my office I give myself once or twice weekly Gentle Wave treatments, and twice yearly Botox injections. That is my complete face-care routine in a nutshell.

If you have a moisturizer you love but it does not have an SPF (such as MD Skin Care daily moisturizer), what do you do?

Use the one you love *and* put an SPF on top of that.

How do you know how much SPF you need daily?

SPF 15 or higher is good. It is important to reapply every two hours, since the SPF degrades with sun exposure.

THE BIG O

Olive oil is nice with bread and on pasta, but did you ever really think it could do wonders for your skin? DHC Olive Virgin Oil ($38, www.dhccare.com) is made from a pure olive oil, which has superior ability to moisturize and soften skin. Use day and night as the final component to your skin care routine and you will see rejuvenation begin.

What are the top skin care treatments for rosacea, a condition that causes ruddy skin?

Laser and intense pulsed light treatments are really helpful. Several treatments are required and maintenance treatments over time are also necessary. It is also important to educate the patient to help them understand and minimize the triggers of rosacea: sun, alcohol, stress, spicy foods.

Are there any daily products like over-the-counter moisturizers that will help calm the redness down?

It's important to use gentle products. Good Skin has a line for red/irritated skin, which includes those with rosacea. I wanted antiaging, emollient, gentle products that would help calm rosacea-type skin. The line includes anti-irritants such as caffeine and plant extracts that are soothing and calming to the skin. The line also has an SPF 25 moisturizer that is fabulous.

Daily Moisturizers

OUTRAGEOUS Naturopathica Crème Cassis Bio Amino Replenishment Cream ($85)

Leading spas and resorts, (800) 669-7618, or www.naturopathica.com

We seriously can't afford this product, but it's seriously good. It's the ultimate skin drink for complexions craving serious hydration minus the heavy, greasy feel of rich moisturizers. This concentrated replenishment cream is fortified with essential plant amino acids like hyaluronic acid and vitamins (C, B, and E) to prevent collagen breakdown, improve connective tissue elasticity, and provide beautiful, nourished skin with a dewy glow. It also contains black currant oil, which supports collagen synthesis.

HIGH MD Skincare Maximum Moisture Treatment ($38)

Nordstrom's, Bergdorf Goodman, Sephora, (888) 830-SKIN, or www.mdskincare.com

The price is almost as high as the brand's ego, but it's still among the best. It works on nearly all skin types, goes on light, and never lets your skin feel dry or irritated.

MILKY WAY

If you want the look of firmer, smoother skin, then add DHC Q10 Milk ($36, www.dhccare.com) to your beauty regimen. It's a milky gel-based moisturizer that brings suppleness back to the skin and it's good for all skin types.

MEDIUM **Olay Total Effects Visible Anti-Aging Vitamin Complex ($18.99)**

Mass retailers

We hate to confuse moisturizers with antiaging products, but this combines the benefits of both. While we are not touting antiaging products in this book—at least not much—we cannot ignore that this moisturizer is just fantastic and happens to also diminish the appearance of fine lines and wrinkles, improve skin tone, smooth skin surface, minimize the appearance of pores, and visibly reduce the appearance of blotches and age spots. Now, if it could only do the laundry!

LOW **Aveeno Positively Smooth Facial Moisturizer ($14)**

Mass retailers

Nearly every member of our panel that works in the skin care industry likes Aveeno. It doesn't have any irritating effects on the skin and absorbs nicely, leaving your skin feeling smooth and supple.

LOW **Olay Complete Daily Illuminating UV Lotion ($13.49)**

Mass retailers

It's taken Ms. Olay a few decades, but now that she has completely reintroduced herself, this creamy debutante has it all: a pampering vitamin-rich complex to enhance the skin's natural radiance.

THE AUTHORS' PICK is the Olay Complete, hands down. Olay just seems to have it all: it feels great on the skin, never clogs pores, and softens without leaving a greasy feeling.

Daily Moisturizers with SPF

Ever had a beautifully brown Thanksgiving turkey, a real image straight from Norman Rockwell and the *Saturday Evening Post*, only to take a bite and find it dry and tough as an old work shoe? What good is being perfectly browned if you're just as dry and leathery? That's why that daily moisturizer with SPF is so important: you can now be protected from the sun until you're a lovely tan, and still remain soft and supple.

OUTRAGEOUS **Bobbi Brown EXTRA SPF 25 Moisturizing Balm ($75)**

www.bobbibrown.com

This is a thick, creamy moisturizer but really packs a punch with the high SPF and lots of do-good ingredients.

HIGH **Olay Complete Defense Daily UV Moisturizer, SPF 30 ($13.49)**

Mass retailers

THE FACE OF LUXURY

The most luxurious face masque available today was once only available to celebrities. It's the Z. Bigatti Total Face Masque, and it retails for $275 for a pack of five. The ingredients are imported from around the world and are a highly coveted secret, according to our insider source.

Let us not forget our words of praise for the Olay product line; that they added SPF 30 in a lightweight product just makes it that much better. As Olay will tell you, skin protection does not have to be heavy. Dermatologists recommend using SPF 15 or higher, depending on individual needs and preferences. Also, whether you are walking to the car or sitting by the window, daily activities put your skin at risk. In fact, on average a person receives eighteen hours of incidental sun exposure each week. The Skin Cancer Foundation recommends Olay Complete Defense SPF 30 as an effective UV sunscreen moisturizer that can help reduce the risk of certain types of skin cancer.

HIGH DHC Rich Moisture ($27)

www.dhccare.com

DHC Rich Moisture is rich in do-good ingredients like olive oil, squalane, ginseng, and royal jelly. It just doesn't get any richer and it's good for most skin types.

MEDIUM Eucerin Sensitive Facial Skin Extra Protective Moisture Lotion ($10)

Mass retailers

Eucerin consistently delivers elegant products at a good price. Our experts tell us that this product works well on all skin types because it was created with sensitive skin in mind.

LOW Clean & Clear Morning Glow Moisturizer with SPF 15 ($5.99)

Mass retailers

If you're one of us, you're thinking "I'm glad I had fun in my twenties, but now I need to be responsible" and the first order of business is good skin protection. From our lips to your ears: this is a wonderful, light moisturizer that seems to work well on all skin types, so quit stallin'.

THE AUTHORS' PICK for Maureen is the Olay, because Olay Complete Defense Daily is the lightest product and gives you the most bang for the buck. Paula, however, loves the Clean & Clear because it is even less expensive than the Olay and never irritates her skin. It's also a very light moisturizer that absorbs quickly.

Tinted Moisturizers

OUTRAGEOUS MD Skincare All-In-One Tinted Moisturizer Sunscreen SPF 15 ($38)

Nordstrom's, Bergdorf Goodman, Sephora, www.mdskincare.com, or (888) 830-SKIN

Don't do so much heavy lifting with your face. This tinted moisturizer contains SPF #15 and adds just a touch of color. We also love it because it's light and works well on every skin type.

CRAVING ALMONDS?

For skin that is very, very dry, add a few drops of almond oil to your moisturizer. This makes whatever you're using very enriching without having to add more product.

OUTRAGEOUS pixi hydrotint duo ($38)

www.pixibeauty.com

This is your passport to perfection, your one makeup product that saves time on everything, and this year's all-around beauty winner. The clever ball at the top looks like plastic, but that's the lip and cheek tint and—like Willy Wonka's Everlasting Gobstopper—it seems that no matter how many times you use it for a fresh flush of color, it never gets smaller. Twist off the top and there's your tinted moisturizer with SPF 20, and it's packed with antioxidants. They really should have called it the pixi hydrotint quadruple.

HIGH Tarte Smooth Operator ($35)

www.sephora.com

What do New York fashion editors and Saudi princesses have in common? Answer: Tarte Smooth Operator. We know, we asked (ah, yes, we do have friends in the Saudi royal family, so there!). For a foundation with SPF 20, this one really packs a punch because it's so lightweight and smooth. It also never cakes.

NEUTROGENA MOISTURE OIL-FREE FORMULA, SPF 15 ($10)

Mass retailers

If you find yourself lost in a sea of ever-expanding moisturizers, you cannot beat the Neutrogena brand in this category for the price. It's nongreasy and gives just the right amount of tint for a healthy glow without the heavy feeling of a foundation.

THE AUTHORS' PICK here was a tough decision. Frankly, we love the MD Skincare. It goes on light, never irritates, and lasts the day. The only problem is, who can afford it? Dr. Gross, we implore you, please make a version for the budgets of mere mortals!

Night Creams

While you're sleeping your skin is building the strength to make it through tomorrow. Knowing this, don't you want to nourish your skin while you're sleeping, give it that extra boost it needs to put in the late shift?

HIGH Lancôme Hydra Zen Night ($50)

Fine department stores

If a night of excessive square dancing and bobbing for apples leaves your skin tired and dry, this night treatment is a stroke of genius for your skin. It's thick and does the trick.

MEDIUM Olay Regenerist Continuous Night Recovery ($18.99)

Mass retailers

This nighttime cream does an impressive rendition of midnight serenade while it prepares your skin for the boardroom jungle. Olay Regenerist

LEEPING BEAUTY

can't live off the canvas forever and nighttime is the best time to renew the layers beneath the sur- . DHC Extra Nighttime Moisture ($30, www.dhccare.com) is an intensive moisture treatment forti- with collagen so your skin gets back a little firmness with each passing night.

Continuous Night Recovery was specifically cre-ated to make the most of your slumber with Olay Amino-Peptide Complex (which includes vitamins and green tea extract).

LOW NIVEA Visage Multiple Results All in One Anti-Aging Treatment Night Serum Concentrate ($14.99)

Mass retailers

It's a mouthful, but it really does something won-derful as you sleep. Smooth all over your face and neck at night after cleansing and toning, and your fine lines and wrinkles are visibly reduced, your skin is firmer and smoother, your pores are more refined, and the appearance of your skin tone is evened out. At $14.99 this is the best antiaging beauty buy in our book!

THE AUTHORS' PICK is the NIVEA Visage. It's so thick and creamy and you wake up with skin that is so plump, soft, and refreshed you want to go back to bed in fear you'll mess it up during the day.

Straight Talk About Skin

Eden Grimaldi, an uber-beauty publicist and owner of Media Craft in New York City with a client roster that reads like the Who's Who in beauty products, came to us with her client skyn ICELAND and asked us if we were ad-dressing the issue of stressed skin in our book. "What exactly *is* stressed skin?" we asked. Here are the answers from skyn ICE-LAND's stressed skin expert, Diane C. Mad-fes, M.D., a dermatologist, and clinical instructor at Mt. Sinai Medical Center in New York City.

What causes skin to be stressed?

The cells in our skin are constantly regenerat-ing to maintain a protective barrier between us and the world. When our bodies are exposed to stress, this barrier breaks down. Stress trig-gers a release of adrenalin and other hormone mediators (such as cortisol and histamine) into the bloodstream, triggering a cascade of reactions. Both internal and external stressors

SKYN SOLUTIONS

From our perspective here at *Beauty Buyble* central, if you're not totally buying the stressed skin thing, but you think your skin is definitely in need of a break, try the Skyn ICELAND 5 Day Detox Kit for Stressed Skin ($45, www.skyniceland.com) as a kick start. The kit is a compact, easy-to-tote com-panion for the home or on the road. It contains Glacial Face Wash, a creamy foaming cleanser that re-freshes and purifies chronically stressed skin; Arctic Face Mist, a boost of instant, cooling relief for irritated or inflamed skin; and ANTIDOTE Quenching Daily Lotion, a hydrating tonic for chronically stressed skin. And finally, Oxygen Infusion Night Cream dramatically fortifies and energizes the skin overnight to improve tone and texture.

create an inflammatory reaction throughout our bodies, which causes the formation of free radicals. Free radicals, if unchecked, damage cell membranes, lipids, and proteins in the skin. A buildup of free radicals can lead to skin aging and trigger flare-ups of underlying skin disorders.

How does stress manifest itself on the skin? What are the symptoms?

There are many manifestations of stress on the skin. Most commonly it is in the form of acne breakouts. Acne is caused by the production of sebum or oils from sebaceous glands. Sebaceous glands have receptors or "on/off switches" on their surface and during times of stress, adrenaline and other inflammatory mediators (or "signals") turn on these switches. This reaction is known as androgen up regulation.

Other skin conditions are also negatively affected by stress. Specific signals or neurotransmitters correlate to different diseases; two examples are psoriasis and hives. Our sensory nerves release neuropeptides that cause local inflammation in the skin.

Symptoms of this inflammatory response can be seen with worsening of an underlying skin condition, such as acne, rosacea, psoriasis, or eczema, and as the facial skin begins to look sallow or dull.

How do you know if your skin is stressed?

The effects of internal and external stress take a toll on your skin. The skin's regeneration process slows down and our protective barrier is no longer intact, causing us to be more sensitive to external factors. The skin looks tired and inflamed, and the skin surface becomes dull and/or ruddy, causing it to look blotchy and uneven.

What is the best way to deal with stressed skin?

The best way is to take a deep breath and try to relax, which helps to decrease the adrenalin surge. But this is just the starting point. The inflammatory cascade has already been activated. Applying topical antioxidants and natural soothers will decrease the response. Antioxidants are substances that protect cells from this "oxidative" stress. Antioxidants scavenge and eliminate free radicals. Addi-

WINNING SKIN FROM WITHIN

You can now drink your way to beautiful skin or suck on a candy for the same benefits. How, you ask? Scott Vincent Borba has created the first neutraceutical skin balancing water, BORBA Skin Balance Water ($4 or $60 for a case, www.sephora.com) and BORBA Skin Balance Confections to improve your skin from the inside out. Basically, BORBA water and confections are pumped with super-concentrated vitamins and minerals to increase absorption into the skin. The confections come in gummy and jellybean formulas. . . . mmmmm, yum!

tionally, antioxidants prevent the buildup of further production of other inflammatory mediators, allowing the skin to heal itself.

Eating a well-balanced diet and sticking to a proper skin care regimen are also recommended.

Why is skyn ICELAND good for stressed skin?

skyn ICELAND is the perfect antidote for stressed skin because the line takes some of nature's most nurturing resources and enhances them with the most advanced science to create products that help relieve, heal, and replenish chronically stressed skin.

The line contains many natural antioxidants that attack free radicals and calm down the inflammatory response, which causes premature aging. These antiinflammatories help to immediately reduce redness and irritation created by stress hormones (such as histamine).

skyn ICELAND's proprietary Biospheric Complex delivers the unmatched purity and vital nutrients of Iceland's natural resources to help replenish the key nutrients, such as water and oxygen that are depleted from the skin due to chronic stress. Sourcing ingredients from Iceland, known for its healing and curative waters, skyn ICELAND helps to bring skin back into balance and harmony. For example, white willow bark, a key ingredient in the core prod-

ucts, is a natural antibacterial that helps prevent breakouts and shorten the breakout cycle.

skyn ICELAND transforms exhausted, irritated, and depleted skin so it emerges soft, clear, fresh, and glowing. Incorporating these products in your daily skin care routine should prevent the negative effects of chronic stress on the skin.

Foundation

Everything needs a good foundation. Your house certainly requires a good foundation. Your relationship should have had one, but well, things happen. Your makeup needs a good foundation as well, so that you can build your look with confidence.

All-Day Foundations

Men have great luck with foundations. Look at the Coliseum—it's a sports stadium that has lasted for nearly two thousand years. Now that's a foundation that was built to last. We women, however, would be happy with a foundation that just lasted for a day and perhaps into the evening without making us look cracked and smudged. There is just nothing better than that, but they're harder to find than a good man who is single, employed, straight, and not a total bastard. We have scoured the

EXPERT TRICK

To keep your foundation fresh, refrigerate it. It also helps cool you down when you apply it in warm weather!

options out there and found several good all-day foundations, but unlike the Coliseum, you cannot just take these foundations for granite.

Liquid Foundation

HIGH Chanel Teint Naturel ($57.50)
www.sephora.com

Signs You Have Celeb Potential

1. You never get up before noon.
2. Your dinner parties always have a VIP area.
3. Your favorite words are "fabulous," "chic," and "amazing."
4. You think personal tragedies always happen to other people
5. You wear Chanel Teint Naturel liquid foundation when working out.
6. You have to take a weekend getaway to Ibiza to recoup from an exhausting week of partying.
7. You're on first-name terms with Charlize, Jenn, Angelina, and Brad.

HIGH DHC Velvet Skin Coat ($20)
www.dhccare.com

You will be ready for prime time in no time. Velvet Skin is an invisible primer that fills in any rough patches, ridges, fine lines, and depressions to give you an even, smooth canvas for makeup application. Once you try it you'll wonder what you ever did without it.

MEDIUM Versace Long Lasting and Natural Finish Make-Up ($36)
www.nycbeautybliss.com and www.douglas.de

It is truly disappointing that Versace has discontinued beauty distribution in the United States, because this is the best foundation available. We encourage you to take the extra steps to find it. Try the websites listed. No matter how hard you search, it will be well worth it.

MEDIUM Make Up For Ever Matte Velvet Oil-Free Foundation SPF 20 ($36)
www.makeupforever.com

Forever is a mighty long time, then again looking great forever is a great deal! Why not splurge for a foundation that stays with you?

LOW Revlon Age Defying Makeup with Botafirm ($12.99)
Mass retailers

You can't beat a foundation that goes on effortlessly and looks fresh for up to sixteen hours. Revlon says that this is an unprecedented formula composed of porous polymers and soft silicone, which means that the foundation blends into your skin seamlessly with no caking or clumping. All twelve shades come with a built-in SPF 15.

THE AUTHORS' PICK is the Versace. Hands down, we haven't found another foundation that so cleanly matches skin tones and literally makes anyone's complexion appear flawless.

FOUNDATION FOR SUCCESS

Make Up For Ever professional makeup artist Careth Whitchurch gives the following tips on applying flawless foundation:

➤ The condition of the skin will greatly affect the final outcome of the foundation. Address any dry areas and then prep skin with Make Up For Ever's Corrective Make-up Base ($22), a primer that will minimize fine lines and pores, seal in moisturizer, and create a smoother texture for all skin types. For oily skin, dab a little Make Up For Ever Stop Shining Corrector ($14) on the nose and forehead as well.

➤ Proceed to the foundation of your choice. Adapt your application methods according to the consistency of the foundation. For sheer to medium coverage, Make Up For Ever has developed Face and Body Foundation ($37) and an accompanying Ellipse Sponge ($11), a silk blend reusable beveled sponge specifically designed for the foundation. For more coverage in the areas you need it most, apply in layers or sponge on a little extra and then buff. When using a thicker liquid foundation, such as Liquid Lift or Matte Velvet, a foundation brush and a light touch is just the thing to evenly cover the face.

➤ Apply concealer after foundation for better coverage, and mix in a little Make Up For Ever Metalizer ($19) with your foundation for a healthy glow that will brighten up the face, enhancing the flawless look of the foundation.

Cream Foundations

HIGH shu uemura Velvet Perfect Adjusting Powdery Foundation SPF 14 ($45)

Select fine stores or www.shuuemura.com

There's no denying the simple appeal of a duo (foundation to powder and back), but few beauty brands get it right, without the final results being too clumpy or bumpy. This perfect twosome has it all in one simple compact. Too bad it's so expensive.

MEDIUM Mary Kay Dreamy Creme-to-Powder Foundation ($14)

www.marykay.com

There are very few dual-functioning foundations that actually live up to their claims, but this is one that does. It glides on like a cream when the pad is wet and gives a flawless foundation. Then, go back for powder touch-ups with a dry pad and you will find perfect results here, too.

LOW Maybelline Dream Matte Mousse ($9)

Mass retailers

Maybelline Dream Matte Mousse is so creamy and dreamy we just can't stop touching it. We love the way it feels, glides over the skin, and doesn't feel greasy.

THE AUTHORS' PICK is the Maybelline, because the creamy texture glides on and blends elegantly into your skin without looking heavy. And for the price, the Maybelline outperforms most of the more expensive foundations.

QUICK TIP Celebrity makeup artist Troy Surratt, whose clients include Leann Rimes, Hilary Swank, Charlize Theron, Mandy Moore, the Olsen twins, Cynthia Nixon, and Kate Capshaw, advises that you should always use your fingers to apply foundation in order to get the most natural finish—especially Maybelline's Dream Matte Mousse, because the warmth of your hands helps to melt the product. "I don't usually recommend sponges, because they soak up the product and you run out of it faster. The finish is also simply not as natural."

Stick Foundations

Have you ever been one of "those girls" who has used lipstick for blush? Shame on you. No, really. Shame on you. Yet, what was the siren's song that lead you to sin against beauty so heinously that you opted to look like a clown? For most women, they were just out of rouge (hopefully). However, the ease of using a stick to add a little color without the mess of powder or liquid base is very tempting. There are now a proliferation of quality stick bases which provide convenience and cleanliness for the woman on the go, and now you get these benefits without looking positively dopey.

HIGH BECCA Stick Foundation ($40)
Fine salons or www.sephora.com

Recently, our dear friend Carolyn wrote to us with these ten steps to nabbing a jet-set tycoon. She explained that she herself successfully applied them and wanted to share her tips with us. We were gob-smacked to find that one of her tricks involved using the BECCA Stick foundation. Who knew?

TEN STEPS TO NABBING A JET-SET TYCOON:

➤ Scrub up: do a head to toe reevaluation of your wardrobe, wax, buff, and polish.

➤ Follow the money: head to Ibiza, Cannes, or Monaco.

➤ Don't forget to pack your BECCA Stick Foundation; it takes ten years off and will help you nab your captain of industry.

➤ Talk the talk; bone up on the film industry, particularly the Indies.

➤ Laugh at all his jokes, he'll never know you're faking it.

➤ Return every other phone call, you want to be laid-back but intrigued all the same.

➤ Look like a million dollars at all times.

➤ Be mysterious—jet black eyeliner adds to the mystery.

➤ Flirt with other men—it will make him crazy.

➤ Grasp every opportunity—your mission is 24/7, and opportunity may only come around once.

HIGH MAC Studio Stick SPF 15 ($27)
www.maccosmetics.com

The poolside daybeds at Caesar's Palace Hotel & Casino are flanked with thick white curtains that you can lower when things heat up. But be warned: you will have to get to the bed and back without being in the shade. Your MAC Studio Stick with SPF 15 will make sure you're covered, and with fifteen different shades, this is a foundation stick that just can't be beat. The creamy, smooth stick foundation gives a natural flaw-free

NO ROSY GLOW

Anyone who sufferes from rosacea or reddening of the skin on the face will thank us for this little tip. Benefit's "You're Bluffing!" ($20) is a buttermilk-yellow cream stick that covers up that flush. There's also a bluff puff ($20) that goes hand in hand with the bluff dust ($22) if you're feeling hot under the collar. Dust away redness while you gather your cool.

finish, and the stick has easy twist-up action. The application is precise and fast. You'll want to stick with this one.

LOW Black Opal Crème Stick Foundation ($8.95)
Drugstores

Don't leave your style to chance; eliminate the flaws with this creamy stick foundation that goes on effortlessly. You'll be so put together you'll give 'em all a run for their money.

THE AUTHORS' PICK is the BECCA, because it comes in a wide variety of shades that blend easily with nearly all skin tones and sets up like a liquid foundation, without caking the way so many stick foundations do. It's also great for quick touch-ups.

Foundations For Dark Complexions

HIGH Three Custom Color Specialists ($65 and up)
www.threecustom.com

This is a truly unique company, specializing in custom-blending for any skin type or tone. The challenge with the foundation is that the custom blending must be done on a one-on-one basis, in person, at their New York City location. However, they do have some ready-to-wear concealers you can choose from on their website that start at $36.50 for a single compact and $19.50 for each additional compact of that shade at the time of your order. Just mail a sample of your concealer (or even a discontinued shade you love) in a plastic baggie with your shipping/billing address and a contact number and they will create the shade you want. Your personal "recipe" will remain permanently in the Three Custom Color Specialists' archives for future reorders.

MEDIUM Mary Kay Foundation ($14)
www.marykay.com

The sheer, flawless finish can't be beat and the pigments are strong and varied for even the darkest skin tones. It also comes in coverage for normal-to-oily skin and normal-to-dry skin.

LOW Black Opal Oil-Free Liquid Foundation ($8.65)
Drugstores and discount stores

"Black opal is my favorite foundation," says Tasha Turner, beauty editor for *Essence* magazine. "It's lightweight and comes in a wide range of colors for darker skin tones. I don't leave my house without it, and I suggest you do the same."

THE AUTHORS' PICK is the Black Opal, because it comes in such a wide range of col-

DYNAMIC DUOS
Black Radiance cosmetics has new, captivating eye shadow compacts with two hues for contouring and shading called Dynamic Duo Eye Shadow ($2.99, mass retailers). These velvety powders glide on smoothly and are crease-resistant. We love Fire/Desire and Vintage/Retro.

ors and goes on as well as many of the more expensive brands. It also lasts the entire day without streaking or creasing.

MAKEUP TIPS

Trae Bodge, cofounder of Three Custom Color Specialists (www.threecustom.com), offers the following advice on finding the right shade for your concealer and foundation, no matter what your skin shade.

➤ Finding the perfect shade of concealer for any skin tone is a challenge, but it should be a priority if you wear makeup!

➤ When shopping for a concealer or foundation, trying it on the skin before you buy is vital.

And when you try it on, the best light to view it in is daylight; standard department store lighting often distorts color. If you can, step outside the store for a moment with a mirror. If this is not possible, see if you can find a halogen light in the beauty department—it gives off a light very close to daylight.

➤ For foundation in particular, or any concealer that you plan to use on broad areas of the face, a good place to test a shade is along the jawline. The color you choose should definitely match there, as you want to avoid any demarcation between the neck and jaw.

➤ There are so many uses for concealer that you should try the right shade where you plan

AFRICAN AMERICAN BEAUTY—TOP TO BOTTOM

Tasha Turner, beauty editor for *Essence* magazine, shares her favorites: "These are the products that soothe, revive, nourish, and color me from head to toe."

➤ I trade shampoos regularly because my scalp is dry and flaky, and change is key. I usually cleanse with Nioxin because dandruff shampoos are stripping and drying to the hair (African American hair is dry to begin with). I follow this with a moisturizing shampoo. Anything by Ojon is my favorite; their conditioner and hair masks work wonders. The palm nut oil formula hydrates my hair and gives it a smooth, frizz-free finish without my having to manipulate my hair with a lot of heat styling.

➤ Because of my job as a beauty editor, I have to sample a ton of products. I am a true believer in facials, and my favorites are the Clarins Hydrating Facial Treatment and Glycolic Peels at the Skin Clinic. At home I love the Erno Lazlo System. It completely clears up any breakouts. My other favorites are Clarins Intense Moisture moisturizer and the entire Dermalogic system, which helps to hydrate my skin after the long winter months.

➤ My skin is pretty even-tone, so I don't wear a lot of coverage. My process: Amazing Cosmetics concealer, Cover Girl tinted moisturizer, Dior Eyeliner (brown), and Scott Barnes or Armani Bronzer, which gives me a great glow during the summer and winter months. I am a diehard lip gloss girl. My favorites right now are MAC Oh Baby, Clinique Peach Goddess, and Armani Lip Shimmer # 19.

to use it, such as under the eyes to address circles, around the nose to address redness, on blemishes or scarring, and so on. Some women are fortunate enough to be able to use one concealer for all these issues, but there are others who may need more than one shade, as these issues can sometimes require more aggressive concealing. It is common for African American women to have very dark eye circles, which requires a different approach than, say, redness around the nose. Overall, the goal with concealer and foundation is that your skin should look uniform after applying.

➤ More and more brands are making colors for women of all skin tones, and these are the brands you should seek out. If you approach a counter and see three shades, move on to a counter that has more shades. When designing our collection of concealers, it was very important to us to have a broad range to accommodate women of all skin tones, so we created ten shades. Other great brands that have a broad range of shades for women of color are MAC and Bobbi Brown. Also seek out specific brands for women of color.

➤ If you're tired of searching, the ultimate way to find the right color is to have one custom-blended! We offer this service, as does Prescriptives. If you have found your skin to be a tough match, have a color blended just for you.

CHRISTIAN BRETON MAKEUP LINE

Christian Breton, one of the greatest names in French cosmetics since its introduction in 1991, has recently launched its complete makeup collection in the United States. Christian Breton is a multiethnic line made up of an endless palette of shades, so no matter what age or skin type, all women will find the most suitable colors to further enhance their beauty.

➤ Christian Breton foundations range from pale white to chocolate brown, with textures varying according to the intensity of the shade to suit every skin type.

➤ The liquid foundation is absorbed rapidly by the skin and has a matte finish. It is specially formulated for long-lasting, heavier coverage.

➤ The cream foundation is solid and creamy, and melts upon contact with the skin, where it changes to a light powdery film. It gives the skin a semimatte finish and light coverage.

➤ Christian Breton powders are silky to touch and give a smooth, even finish. They come in loose and pressed.

➤ Christian Breton Terra Tan Sun Powder is made of ultrafine light texture that is created by mixing the powder with silicones in tin tanks, shaping them, and placing them on biscuit trays to bake for twenty-four hours. The "cookies" are then placed in a dryer overnight, and the result is an extraordinarily light and glossy bronzing powder.

MAKEUP TIPS FOR ASIAN WOMEN

San Francisco–based makeup artist Reiko Kobayashi shares her favorite products and offers the following makeup tips for Asian faces:

➤ Foundation: Giorgio Armani's Luminous Silk Foundation is great for every face, especially for Asian complexions. It's a silicone-based foundation with a light to medium coverage that gives a great glow to the skin ($52.50). Apply it using Armani's foundation brush for a flawless finish ($53.50). giorgioarmani.com

➤ Concealer: YSL's Touche éclat sheer, multi-purpose concealer camouflages dark circles and highlights the eye area. It can also be used as a shadow base ($36). Nordstrom.com

➤ Highlighter: Giorgio Armani's Fluid Sheer comes in several shades for all types of skin tones. For the dewy luminous look, apply #0, #2, or #7 fluid sheer on the cheekbones using Giorgio Armani's foundation brush ($52.50). giorgioarmani.com

➤ Powder: Giorgio Armani's Silk Foundation Powder is a great powder to set your foundation. Apply using a powder brush and dust all over the face. ($46). giorgioarmani.com

➤ Lips: YSL Rouge Pur # 121 lipstick can be used alone without a lip liner for that cute pouty lip ($26). Nordstrom.com

➤ Blush: NARS Amour blush. Gorgeous on Asian skin tones ($22). beauty.com

➤ Eye Shadow: Chanel's Variation Quadra eye shadow ($55). Nordstrom.com

➤ Eyeliner: Bobbi Brown's Gel Eyeliner in black ($18). Nordstrom.com

➤ Eyeshadow Brush: Chanel's Shadow/Liner Brush ($18.50). Nordstrom.com

➤ Mascara: YSL's Lengthening and Curling Mascara ($24). Nordstrom.com

USE THESE PRODUCTS TO CREATE A GREAT LOOK FOR ASIAN EYES:

➤ Apply the almond eyeshadow shade all over the eyelid. Apply the caramel shade below the browbone. Apply the toast over the caramel shade.

➤ Using all four colors from the variation palette—mousse, toast, almond, caramel—build the colors by layering, then blending.

➤ Using the gel eyeliner, draw a medium-thick line across your upper lash line. Then, apply the mousse eyeshadow over the eyeliner using short, upward strokes. The Chanel shadow/liner brush is perfect for blending the mousse on lower lash line.

BRONZING POWDER

We thought face bronzing was one of the oldest tricks in the game, but 1984, when Guerlain created the first bronzing powder, is not really that long ago. Today, Guerlain Terracotta is an indispensable bronzer that has become the benchmark for all bronzers. It retails for $36 and is available at fine department stores such as Neiman Marcus, Saks Fifth Avenue, and Bergdorf Goodman.

➤ Apply YSL lengthening and curling mascara and let it dry.

➤ Gently curl lashes with Trish McEvoy's eyelash curler.

Face Powders

Pressed Face Powder

It's the face powder that's pressed, not powders for a pressed face. Pressing will do little to help your face from a cosmetic standpoint, unless you're going for that English bulldog look. Pressed face powders, however, can be a tremendous help as you beautify.

HIGH CAT Cosmetics Cat Call Powder ($24)

www.catcosmetics.com

Put down the dice, back away from the table, and say pshaw to the pool. With Cat Call Powder you can roll the dice anywhere, any time, because it won't leave you even if you think there's a chance of shine-through. With Cat Call Powder, you always strike a purrfect tone and cause all the guys to paws and reflect on your magnificence. It will always leave you feline fine, and you never have to worry about looking like kitty litter.

HIGH Benefit Georgia, and Dandelion ($26)

www.benefitcosmetics.com

Georgia is a concoction of peaches 'n' cream that's perfect for blondes. It will give your face a delightfully warm glow. Dandelion gives the sheer softness of pink—perfect for brunettes—for a sweet and irresistible matte finish. You can use them over foundation or alone.

LOW Sally Hansen CornSilk Shineless Matte ($5.50)

Mass retailers

CornSilk is a grandmother's staple, but why? Because it works, that's why. The corn silk is particularly great for oily or acne-prone skin because it absorbs oils more effectively, which lifts the dirt and oil away from the skin. It also reduces the appearance of pore size and contains walnut shell powder, which is just plain interesting, don't you think?

e.l.f. Clarifying Pressed Powder ($1)

www.elfcosmetics.com

We cannot ignore the allure of $1 beauty products that behave like a million dollars. We have to assume that anyone who would know of such a brand would buy this one first, but we didn't know about e.l.f. until we sat down to write this book, and now we're hooked. The Champs Elysee

POWDER PANDEMONIUM

Oops! You now have loose powder on your clothes, or is that the deodorant mark from this morning? Not sure? No problem. Miss Oops Rescue sponges will save the day. Briskly rub the dry sponge against the offending mark and watch it disappear. The patent-pending sponges come two to a pack, are safe to use on all fabrics, and are reusable ($10, www.missoops.com).

Tower suite seems like an unlikely place to whip out your e.l.f, but it's not. It stops the shine, helps prevent breakouts, and has a shielding hydra-tint of SPF 15, so why wouldn't you want to flaunt it?

THE AUTHORS' PICK is split: Maureen loves the e.l.f. because she feels both chic and thrifty when she uses it, and Paula loves the CAT because it's not too thick, never clumps, and comes in so many different shades that everyone can be accommodated.

FAB FACE IN FIFTEEN MINUTES

For all you girls on the go, celebrity makeup artist Jacqueline Shepherd tells us how to get glam in just fifteen minutes flat.

➤ Cleanse face with Soy Cleanser from Fresh. It's pefect for those of us too lazy to remove eye makeup first because it's gentle but does the job quickly.

➤ Apply a moisturizer with sunscreen (Murad tinted sunscreen with pomegranate is my favorite).

➤ Use a concealer under the sides of nose and any discolored/red area. I love Stila concealers because they have a great consistency and retain moisture. For dark circles, try Paula Dorf EyeLite eye brightening stick or Benefit ohh la lift!

➤ Apply your foundation mixed with a dab of highlighting elements, such as MAC strobe cream or golder shimmer. This adds opalescence, vibrancy, and youthful glow.

➤ Using fingertips dab a pink or peach cream blush to the apples of your cheeks and blend till the outside of a possibly clownish circle disappears into the skin. This will make any woman of any age look flushed and healthy.

➤ Put just a swipe of NARS Orgasm blush over cream blush to keep the cream blush in place.

➤ Curl lashes. Try Benefit BAD gal lash mascara for supple, full, and moist lashes. Always brush lashes *up and away* from the corners to open up the eyes.

➤ Use your fingertips to dab some Navajo gold cream shadow from Bodyography on your

CELEBRITY POWDER TIP

Makeup artist Rebecca Restrepo, whose cadre of celebrity faces includes Julia Stiles, Mary Louise Parker, and Anna Paquin, loves the Kevyn Aucoin loose face powder: "It doesn't collect and make you look old the way so many that are too thick do." Rebecca's application tips: for a finish that will last all day, apply with a powder puff, sponge, or even a synthetic brush because they hold the powder more to the skin. For a light finish, use the natural bristle brush. For more opaque coverage, pat it on with the sponge. Don't use your fingers; the grease on your fingers won't allow you to set the powder properly. Fingers work when applying foundation because the oils help you manipulate the product, keeping it thinner and looking more like skin, but this doesn't work with powder.

lids, and a quick swipe of the Bodyography Orgasm blush over the gold cream blush.

➤ Choose a nice soft neutral lip gloss for daytime. For those on the plumping train, try LipFusion in Bare. Yes, it does work, they say in forty-eight hours—it's more like four hours—but who cares? Reapply, baby!

Loose Face Powder

There are times that call for cutting loose. A loose face powder is ideal when you want a sheer coverage, nothing too cakey or clumped.

OUTRAGEOUS Kevyn Aucoin Gossamer Loose Powder ($62)

www.kevynaucoin.com

This is a superfine powder that provides an always-fresh look and comes with the unique Kevyn Aucoin cellulose sponge applicator. Celebrity makeup artists love this product and, despite the outrageous price, you'll be hooked, too. It comes in two shades: Diaphanous, which is a pearly shade and Radiant Diaphanous, which is slightly tinted for darker skin tones.

HIGH Jurlique Rose Silk Dust ($25)

www.jurlique.com to find a retailer near you

Like fairy dust, Jurlique Rose Silk Dust is so light and velvety you won't even notice it. Yet, it provides a matte finish that is sheer and natural without clumping or flaking.

LOW Sally Hansen CornSilk Shineless ($5.49)

Mass retailers

Never underestimate a good walnut. Walnuts apparently have many benefits, the most important of which is found in the Sally Hansen CornSilk

face powder our mothers used. It's also in the product that sits on drugstore shelves today. The secret to the success of CornSilk is the walnut shell powder, a superfine powder that is known for its oil-absorbing properties. The walnut shell powder also gives the CornSilk its silky feel and sheer effect, and it blends with most any skin color. The No Color shade is good for darker skin tones.

THE AUTHORS' PICK is the Jurlique Rose Silk Dust because it goes on like silk, and you never have that heavy cakey feeling you get from a lot of face powders. There's also a subtle shimmer to it, so you'll glow.

Concealers

Blemish Concealers

We all have things we want to conceal: our income, our weight, our age, and the fact that we think the trainer at the local gym is better looking than the man in our lives. Concealers can hide a huge number of sins, so having a good concealer is very important. Sticks should be used with care. You don't want to swipe them across your face so hard that you pull on your skin, or you'll just contribute to wrinkling. Instead, dab and blot or place it on your fingertips and then apply gently, blending as you go.

OUTRAGEOUS Three Custom Color Specialists ($36.50)

www.threecustom.com

We've discussed Three Custom Color Specialists earlier in the book. Because we think they're so important, we're going to follow the age-old shampoo doctrine and apply it to concealer: brain-wash, rinse, and repeat. Where else can you get your own personal recipe in a concealer that's rich, creamy, and doesn't irritate the skin? We rest our case.

HIGH Dermablend Quick-Fix Concealer ($17–$28)
Mass retailers or www.dermablend.com

This is a megaconcealer that you can use to cover dark under-eye circles, fine lines, age spots, blemishes, or even a scar. If you have serious pigmentation to cover, this is your product. It's not exactly lightweight, but if it was good enough for the cast of *Sex and the City,* you're sure to love the results if you're in need of some high coverage. It's also smudge-resistant, water-resistant, and lasts up to sixteen hours.

LOW Max Factor Erase ($5)
Mass retailers

Don't know about you, but we certainly have a few skeletons from our past we'd love to erase. But that could take some time, so for quick touch-ups on marks, blemishes, or bumps you actually can conceal, this oldie but goodie can't be beat.

e.l.f. Tone Correcting Concealer ($1)
www.elfcosmetics.com

Fresh from prison, Martha Stewart came out looking younger and slimmer. The former is due to well-placed concealer, and just goes to show how much it can do to resurrect a tired face. Just think what Martha might say about this concealer for only $1. Now that's a good thing!

THE AUTHORS' PICK is the e.l.f. because it glides on, hides most flaws with just the right amount of coverage, and never cakes.

APPLYING CRÈME CONCEALER
Here's advice from Trae Bodge, cofounder of Three Custom Color Specialists, on how to apply crème concealer:

Because concealers come in so many different formulations, it's tough to advise on an application that covers each type of formulation. Three Custom Color Specialists carries a crème concealer formula, so I'll provide application tips for crèmes:

➤ For isolated areas, such as the eyes, around the nose, or for blemishes, I recommend a brush for application. The brush should be no larger than ½ inch wide, have synthetic bristles (best suited for wet products), and taper in at the tip, allowing you to get into tiny areas, such as the corners of the eyes and under the lash line. Apply where you need the most coverage and blend outward with tiny strokes.

DERMABLEND REMOVER
Given that Dermablend is the market leader in concealment cosmetics, we recommend the Dermablend remover for all Dermablend makeup products. While traditional makeup removers and soap will work, the Dermablend remover is engineered to break down and remove Dermablend cosmetics quickly, and it's non-abrasive for sensitive skin ($15, www.dermablend.com).

➤ If you wear foundation, apply it over the concealer and set it with powder. If you're not wearing foundation, apply the powder directly over concealer to set.

➤ If you're using the concealer on broader areas of the face, use a larger synthetic bristle brush (1 inch or wider) or a wet or dry sponge. Follow application tips above.

Under-Eye Concealers

You may have spent all night working on a project, but when it comes time for the presentation, you still need to look like you luxuriated through twelve hours of beauty sleep, not like Rocky Balboa after fifteen rounds with Apollo Creed. With a good under-eye concealer, they'll never know that you're dying to curl up on the conference table and take a nap.

HIGH   Bobbi Brown Creamy Concealer Kit ($32) for the kit, or ($22) for the concealer alone

www.bobbibrowncosmetics.com

This creamy concealer is the most powerful for serious dark circles, and combined with the sheer-finish loose powder it's a dynamic duo that can't be beat. It even comes with a mini-powder puff (which is why we recommend the kit and not the concealer alone!).

MEDIUM   Benefit It stick ($18)

www.benefitcosmetics.com

This pencil is the perfect boo-boo eraser and your new best friend. This stick erases everything; red spots, irregular skin marks, pimples, pock marks,

under eye circles, you name it. Just don't count on it for erasing that speeding ticket you're hiding in your bedside drawer.

LOW   Sally Hansen Eye Lifting Gel & Concealer ($5.49)

Mass retailers

This is a great product because it's an antiaging eye lift gel on one end, which gently tightens and smooths the skin under the eye for a "virtual" eye lift, and a concealer on the other end that perfects and brightens.

THE AUTHORS' PICK is the Sally Ha because it solves two problems in one that's a coup when you're trying to be clock every minute of the day.

Mascara

Supposedly, the eyes are the windows to the soul. With that in mind, do you want your eyes to look like the Christmas windows at Sak's Fifth Avenue, or the windows at your local dollar store? What do you think will make the sale? "Eyelashes are the most challenging and delicate area of the eyes," says Dr. Jeffrey Epstein, founder of the Women's Foundation for Hair Loss and the Foundation for Hair in New York City. "The curl and length of your eyelashes is genetically determined, and actually has little relation to the curliness of the scalp hairs."

If the eyes are the window to the soul, the eyelashes are the clapboard shutters that both protect and draw attention to them, so we need to make them pretty, ladies!

Mascara That Lengthens

Give 'em the lash. You want your lashes to be as long and luscious as possible. Of course, we're not all endowed with spectacular lashes. But with a wave of these mascara wands, we can work our magic and create the illusion of long lashes. Think of mascara that lengthens as a Wonderbra for your eyelashes.

HIGH shu uemura Fiber Xtension Mascara ($23)

Department stores and www.sephora.com

This smudge-proof wonder of a mascara lengthens each and every lash evenly, while thickening them at the same time. The result? Mesmerizingly long, luscious lashes.

MEDIUM MAC Zoom Lash ($10)

Unalloyed smarts are not enough. To motivate your man, you need some killer eyelashes, and your eyes will loom impossibly large with MAC Zoom Lash. You'll dazzle him with just one application.

LOW Maybelline XXL Volume + Length Microfiber Mascara ($7.95)

Mass retailers

Although in the low category, this mascara is hardly a third-place finish. This magnificent mascara gives puny lashes a huge boost so you can go from last place to winning look in seconds flat.

FOR THE CAMERA-READY LOOK

Take the lead from Max Factor movie makeup artist Richard Dean, who has painted some of Hollywood's most recognizable faces, including those of Nicole Kidman, Madonna, Demi Moore, Diane Lane, and Glenn Close.

➤ For a classic look, start with a foundation that offers substantial coverage, yet doesn't mask your face's beautiful, natural variations in color. Max Factor Colour Adapt reveals true colors, disguises little imperfections, and offers a delectable finish. Use a sponge, a brush, or your fingers to gently apply—whichever gives you the most comfortable control. Colour Adapt's silky texture makes application a breeze.

➤ A classic eye requires beautiful, yet clean details. Try brushing Max Factor Lasting Colour Eye Shadow in Cameo Appearance across the lid. Then softly contour the lid with Max Factor Lasting Colour Eye Shadow in Fawn by following the natural crease. Along the upper lashes only, line with Max Factor Pensilk in Soft Charcoal.

➤ This classic eye requires a spectacular finish! Nothing will lengthen and dramatize lashes like Max Factor Stretch & Separate Waterproof Mascara. Try curling the lashes, then applying two light coats in Rich Black. Keep the bottom lashes lush and warm with Stretch & Separate Waterproof in Black Brown.

THE AUTHORS' PICK is the Maybelline XXL Volume + Length Microfiber Mascara. We loved the MAC Zoom Lash, but we found comparable effects with the Maybelline product for less money and easier availability.

Waterproof Mascara

Planning on a little pool time? Don't be a frog-woman, think sultry mermaid singing her siren's song to the cabana boys: "Bring me a margarita and the suntan oil."

HIGH shu uemura Mascara Basic ($27)

Fine department stores or www.shuuemura-usa.com

This product comes with a *Beauty Buyble* guarantee: you'll absolutely love it. This mascara not only lengthens, but it's waterproof in a way that's undetectable; it never smears when you go to wash it off. It's amazing.

HIGH Lancôme Définicils Waterproof Mascara ($21.50)

Department stores

Live in Delaware but crave Hollywood? With Lancôme Définicils you'll emerge from the ocean like a goddess with lashes to back it up and mascara intact.

LOW Max Factor Stretch & Separate Waterproof Mascara ($3.50)

Mass retailers

Streamline your life with an old-timer that continues to impress MF brand devotees. This mascara sets out to do what it says through rain or shine.

THE AUTHORS' PICK is the Max Factor Stretch & Separate because it grabs each and every lash and stretches it to the sky, and the price can't be beat.

MASCARA QUICK TIP

MAC celebrity makeup artist Gordon Elliott offers the following tip on creating the most glamorous lash effect. "Before applying mascara, curl your lashes three times. Start as close to the base of the lashes as possible, slide the curler up, curl again about halfway up the length of the lash hairs, and finally curl once more at the tips. This creates a more natural-looking curl to the lashes. Apply mascara in three sections. Brush the inner lashes toward the bridge of the nose, center lashes straight up toward the eyebrow, and finally the outer lashes should be brushed out toward the temple. This technique fans out the lashes, making them look fuller."

EYELASH CURLERS

Our two favorite eyelash curlers are worlds apart—in price, that is. The shu uemura eyelash curler is $16.50 and gives your eyelashes a luscious bend that reaches up to the sky. The e.l.f. eyelash curler is $1 and also takes your lashes to the moon, but for quite a few pennies less.

Fun Mascara

This is an entirely made-up category to satisfy our own desire to throw in some products we love that don't necessarily fit anywhere else.

MEDIUM pixi Duo Lashtint ($22)

www.pixibeauty.com

Our friend Diane was at a party in London when a fashion editor with British *Vogue* grabbed her and said, "What mascara are you wearing?" As Diane relayed it, this was one of those completely chic moments when you've made just the right statement with makeup. "My friends who are writing this very witty and necessary beauty book back in the States turned me on to this lash tint by pixi," she said. "One end has a base color to tint lashes, the other end has a brighter shade to enhance your eye color. I'm wearing black-plum." "I haven't heard of pixi," the British *Vogue* editor responded with shame. Having had years of experience with designer powders, top-flight fix-it face creams, legendary eye shadows, and immaculate lipsticks, Diane was euphoric to finally make the impression she longed for. And for these reasons, we are charged with sharing this double-ended wand, which comes in five color combinations.

pixi Fairy Dust is another beauty staple we've discovered from our pile of pixi. It's holographic fairy dust, which means it reflects light with super metallic texture. And, at $18 a pot, why not?

False Eyelashes

Exercise caution when choosing whether to use false eyelashes. If you know how to apply them and do it correctly, false eyelashes will give you va-va-va-voom and draw attention to your eyes. Applying them incorrectly will also certainly attract attention to your eyes, but not in such a positive light. They will look either like exotic insects trying to escape flypaper, or the brush ends of the attachments to your vacuum cleaner. Neither look is particularly "in" this year.

HIGH MAC Lashes ($9)

Fine stores or www.maccosmetics.com

Beauty-conscious Hollywood types save face with these amazing lashes from MAC because they're so light and fluffy, and let's face it, there's nothing more ultraportable than false eyelashes. Razzle-dazzle 'em with your up-to-the-minute beauty know-how as you apply them at a moment's notice.

MEDIUM Revlon Fantasy Lengths Self Adhesive Maximum Wear Eyelashes ($5.99)

Mass retailers

Don't be surprised if your local drugstore is out of these wonder self-adhesive lashes. They are hotter than being hand fed habañero and Scotch

---

PIXI MUST

You've probably read a bit about pixi products in this book. Our love for pixi runs deep, so we're giving them some more space here for their new pixi Miracle Eye Beauty kit ($28). There are eight glimmering, shimmering shades.

bonnet peppers by an oiled Brad Pitt in a speedo in Death Valley in July.

LOW N.Y.C. Self-Adhesive Eyelashes ($1.99)
Drugstores

If the prospect of paying top dollar for eyelashes you will ultimately discard at the end of the day leaves you cold, appease your inner fussbudget with these perfectly pretty, easy-to-place adhesive eyelashes that you can toss off at their end of your reign without feeling guilty.

THE AUTHORS' PICK is the MAC lashes, because they're simply gorgeous. They feather out like a peacock and give you instant movie star status. Expensive? Yeah. But worth every penny.

Eyebrow Essentials

"Eyebrows are like fingerprints. They vary in shape, length, and thickness. Your brows are unique, so there is no such thing as one brow shape fits all. My mission is to share with you my years of beauty experience, having met and shaped the brows of thousands of beautiful people—both inside and out."

—Love, Eliza

Eliza is known as the Queen of the Arch, and is one of the most influential experts in the beauty industry. She's the waxing director/eyebrow designer at the Avon Salon & Spa in New York City, and she introduced the first-ever salon devoted to brows and beyond. She is on speed dial of her numerous celebrity clients (among them Natasha Richardson, Jennifer Grey, Yasmeen Ghauri, and Tracy Pollan), who affirm that Eliza's skills and knowledge are unsurpassed. She maintains the unique beauty philosophy that it's not just about trimming or tweezing; it's about creating a look, a style, a feeling. Eliza has developed an elegant and efficiently designed kit that includes everything you need to get salon-perfect eyebrows at home, on the run, or wherever your travels take you!

Eliza's Eyebrow Essentials Kit ($68, www.avon.com) is an easy-to-use kit, which includes an eyebrow-sculpting program featuring Eliza's do's and don'ts of eyebrow design. The kit is available in blonde and brunette and includes eight brow-beautiful products used by Eliza herself, along with a comprehensive manual on how to achieve your very own perfect "arch-itechture":

➤ *For Trimming*: **Eliza's Curved Scissors and Dual Brow Brush,** the ultimate weapons against unruly hairs.

THE BEST COLORS FOR DIFFERENT SKIN TYPES

Always take undertone into consideration. For olive undertones, use warmer colors (brown and dark-green) to balance out skin tone. Fair blondes and brunettes with pink undertones usually look best in softer colors, like light blue grays, lavenders, and pale greens. For darker skin, warm and bright colors stand out the best: coppers, yellows, and oranges.

DOUBLE DUTY

Sally Hansen Eye Definers do double duty for eyes with three great eye shadows that go on effortlessly and a crème liner included in a handy four-pack. (www.sallyhansenhealingbeauty.com)

➤ *For Tweezing*: **Eliza's Slanted Tweezers** get a grip on grooming, and **Eliza's Pointed Tweezers** are specially designed to pluck even the most stubborn hair.

➤ *For Finishing*: **Eliza's Brow Definer** is the award-winning pencil that masters any arch; **Eliza's Chunky Brow** is the filler for a fuller brow; and **Eliza's Brow Shaper** is a clear gel that lasts for twenty-four hours to lock in the look.

Eye Shadow

Eye shadow has enormous power. It can make you a sexy, sultry queen of love, or it can make you look like a circus clown. As many women have discovered to their dismay, there is a very fine line between the two and it's the use or misuse of eye shadow that draws the line.

Powder Eye Shadow

HIGH   Chanel Multi-Effects Eyeshadow ($28.50)

Fine department stores

Chanel eye shadow makes every face the picture of perfection. The colors are always the most rich and vibrant, and they seem to continuously hit the mark every year with more powerful shades to choose from than any of their competitors.

MEDIUM   shu uemura Pressed Eye Shadow ($18.00)

Select specialty stores or www.shuuemura.com

As the day wears on, the pressure builds for eye shadow. One thing everyone raves about is that the shu uemura lasts the day without creasing or running, so that you can face the barrage with confidence and always look beautiful.

BEAUTY ADDICTION × 4

Beauty Addicts is our latest addiction. There are four distinct sets of lip, eye, cheek, and sun palettes, with colors that coordinate. *Glow* combines icy pinks and golden bronze shades. *Seduce* plays tribute to the smoky glamour of silvers and blacks. *Express* combines pinks, bronze, gold, and cinnamon tones, and *Motivate* speaks to a sophisticated corporate style with soft pink, lilac, plum and amethyst. Each set is $26–$30, available at www.beautyaddicts.com.

LOW Revlon Eye Shadow ($7)

Mass retailers

We salute the velvety finish of Revlon shadows. They're easily applied with either a fingertip or brush and come in commanding colors to catch the attention of all civilians.

THE AUTHORS' PICK is the Chanel. Sure, it's expensive, but you really look the part in these rich, deep shades that last all day without creasing.

Cream / Liquid Eye Shadow

OUTRAGEOUS Chanel Ombre D'eau Fluid Iridescent Eye Shadow ($30)

Fine stores or (877) 737-4672

The metallic-like finish conjures up images of 1980s Metallica concerts, but what you notice next is how it translates on the eye with an irresistible finish that makes your eyes pop. They come in compelling shades and truly create instant success on the eyes.

HIGH NARS Crème Eye Shadow ($20)

Saks Fifth Avenue, Neiman Marcus, or Sephora stores

The palette may be right, but if you don't have a good cream shadow you'll know it when it finds its way to your chin, and good architecture is only good when it's still standing, right? Our experts love how NARS delivers great shades in soft hues and doesn't fall down on the job.

LOW Almay Color Cream Shadow ($6)

Mass retailers

You finish the "It was so difficult I nearly resigned" project for work, then press the "save" button and the computer crashes. What do you do next? You reach for that oversize chocolate bar you dumped in your bag weeks ago, slide on some Almay Color Cream Shadow, and hit the skids for the nearest bar to meet Mr. Possibly Perfect, knowing that while your day was a disaster, your eyes say, "Come hither, honey," because your shadow is divine.

THE AUTHORS' PICK for Paula is the Chanel Ombre D'eau Fluid Iridescent Eye Shadow because the shades are so divine and it lasts all day. Maureen loves the Almay Color

WATERPROOF EYE SHADOW

We've all seen *The Wizard of Oz.* Do you want to know a secret? When the Wicked Witch of the West screamed, "I'm melting! I'm melting!" it was really because she didn't use waterproof eye shadow. You've all had that Tammy Faye moment when the Botticelli masterpiece face melts into a Picasso in the rain, or when a trollop from Kansas dumps a bucket of cold water over your head. Well, no more. Waterproof eye shadow will keep you looking stunning as you cast the spell to blast that little hussy back to Kansas where she belongs. Now if we could just talk about that green foundation . . .

EYE SHADOW THAT LASTS

If you want your eye shadow to adhere like white on rice, Chanel Professional Eye Shadow Base ($30) is a miracle product. It's lightweight and offers three distinct benefits: it assures longer lasting eye shadow wear, works as an excellent cover-up, and improves the look of your eyes by brightening them like optical pearls.

Cream Shadow. The shades are sophisticated and the cream never creases or bleeds.

Color Stick Eye Shadow

MEDIUM MAC Shadow Shadestick ($15)

www.maccosmetics.com

This is the richest and creamiest eye shadow delivered in a sophisticated stick-style format on the planet. The colors are so potent and rich that others might ask, "Are those gems on your eyes?" The finish is definitely semiprecious and glides on effortlessly. It also works as a shadow or liner for total eye impact.

LOW Sally Hansen Color Stick for Eyes ($4.99)

Drugstores

FUN WITH EYE SHADOW

We fell in love with an irresistible collection of loose cosmetic dusts called Glamo Glitz by Scarlett ($15, www.scarlettcos.com or (800) 862-2311). Here are just a few ways you can use Glamo-Glitz (GG):

➤ *Eye shadow*: Use wet or dry and brush over lid; repeat for a more intense look.

➤ *Eye liner*: Dip an eyeliner brush into water and then into GG, press brush along lash line to define the eye.

➤ *Lips*: Use petroleum jelly on your lips, then mix one part water with two parts GG and dab onto the lips.

➤ *Mascara*: Dip a disposable mascara wand into two parts water with one part GG and sweep along lashes.

➤ *Cheeks*: Dip a blush brush into the GG and dust onto your cheeks.

➤ *Décolleté*: Use a large powder brush to lightly dust GG over your collarbones and anywhere else you desire for a shimmery glow.

The Color Stick for Eyes does double duty as an eyeliner or eye shadow. It glides on smoothly and evenly with no creasing, smudging, or flaking; and the twist-up stick never needs sharpening. Available in twelve shades.

Eyeliners

When you think of big, kohl-rimmed eyes, think Sophie Dahl, Catherine Zeta-Jones, or Angelina Jolie. For full-on Bardot glamour as seen on the catwalk, we recommend a cadre of great eye catchers.

Liquid Eyeliner

Liquid eyeliners can either give you couture eye contour or make you look like an extra from a Tim Burton movie, with dark, semi-melted circles under bloodshot eyes. Mishandling liquid eyeliner doesn't have the extreme consequences of mishandling nitroglycerine, but you still want to be very careful when you apply it, because the results could blow up in your face.

HIGH Bobbi Brown Long-Wear Gel Eyeliner in Black Ink ($18)
Bobbi Brown counters or www.bobbibrown.com

"Say good-bye to eyeliner that ends up everywhere except where you want it to be. . . . Say hello to perfectly lined eyes," says Bobbi Brown. This long-wear gel eyeliner gives you the look of liquid liner with the ease of a gel formula.

MEDIUM MAC Liquid Eyeliner ($11.50)
www.maccosmetics.com or (800) 588-0070

Don't be afraid of going bold around the eyes. Eyeliner can change the collective mood with the sweep of the brush. This eyeliner can take you from dippy to downright deity in seconds flat. We also love that it doesn't run.

LOW Milani Glitter Glamour Duo ($4.99)
Mass retailers

If there is one beauty product that epitomizes our love for bacchanalian debauchery through beauty products, this is the one. This glamour duo has mascara on one end and the grooviest glittery liquid eyeliner on the other in four exciting duos. We are all abuzz over this beauty find, and the price makes us giddy.

Stick Eyeliner

HIGH Sue Devitt Eye Intensifier Pencil ($22)
Barney's New York or (888) 822-7639

Everyone needs structure in their life, and when we start with the eyes there's nothing nicer than a good eyeliner to define the eyes and make them pop. Sue Devitt is a savvy choice because it goes on easily, has a solid yet creamy texture, and comes in ten fantastic shades for every mood.

MEDIUM Cat Cosmetics Eye Pencils ($15)
www.catcosmetics.com

Don't assume that smoky eyes have to be black. If you want that sultry, sexy look, Cat will put the "meow" in your purrrrr. These zippy eye pencils work wonders to transform you from cat to sex kitten.

LOW N.Y.C. Browblender Brow & Liner ($4.99)
Mass retailers

Jet Black and Dark Brown are staple eyeliner colors that also make it easy to line and define brows without the hassle of two separate products. Two pencils come per package, so that's four times the fun!

LOW   e.l.f Brightening Eye Liner ($1)
Mass retailers

It's the gel-powder formula that makes this eyeliner glide on so effortlessly. But what makes us truly nutty about the e.l.f eyeliner is the price. How can it be so good and so cheap? It makes us wonder what the prestige products are really up to.

THE AUTHOR'S PICK is split. Paula loves e.l.f. and Maureen loves Cat, but they both love both so much they don't want to choose. How's that for indecisive?

Waterproof Eyeliner

HIGH   Sue Devitt Eye Intensifier Pencil ($22)
Fine department stores

There is such a thing as gorgeous dishevelment, but you can't have serious sophistication if your eyeliner runs. We love Sue Devitt because it goes on like silk, the shades are rich, and the color never bleeds.

MEDIUM   Too Faced Liquif-Eye ($17.50)
Fine department stores

Just imagine if you could take any of your favorite eye shadows, turn them into eye liner, and ensure they never smudge or budge. Now you can with Liquif-Eye. It's a clear liquid with a felt tip brush that

EYES THAT MAKE A STATEMENT

Make Up For Ever professional makeup artist Careth Whitchurch gives the following tips to make your eyes pop:

➤ When choosing shadow colors, take eye color into consideration. Contrast cool eyes with warm colors and vice versa. For example, for green eyes use purples or coppers; for blue eyes use browns or pinks; for brown eyes use blues and grays. In addition, try highlighting the eye area with a concealer that has light-reflecting particles, like Make Up For Ever's Lift Concealer ($19), which also firms those bags under the eyes.

➤ Remember to curl lashes and for extra "pop," use colored mascara on the bottom lashes to open up the eye.

➤ First date? Subtlety is key. Flawless foundation, understated eyes, and glossy lips are quick and easy ways to do the job! Think pretty, like a soft brown or gray smoky eye with Make Up For Ever's Star Powder #946 or #947 ($17) and flushed cheeks, perfectly achieved with Blush Cream #1. Try Fascinating Lipgloss in #8 ($16) for dazzling natural lips.

TROUBLE WITH BOUNDARIES?

A quick tip from Katherine Hickland, owner and founder of Cat Cosmetics: "Take a soft chocolate brown liner and line just the outer corners of the upper and lower lashline. Then, with a pointy cotton swab, smooth over the line to blur the edge and give you that sexy, smoky look. It really makes the eyes pop."

you use to dip into your eye shadows and then apply as eye liner. The liquification allows you to transform any powder shadow—or even blush for that matter—to eye liner, and the patented liquid seals it on so it's waterproof. Now that's invention!

LOW N.Y.C Waterproof Eyeliner Pencil ($3.99)
Drugstores

You just received an invitation to your father's wedding and your new stepmom is ten years younger than you and half your size. The tears will be rolling down your eyes at the ceremony, but they won't be tears of joy. The last thing you need is your eyeliner to run. Thankfully, N.Y.C. has your back. This eyeliner won't run or smudge, so you can cry all you want and hold your looks well past the reception.

EYELINER NOTES
New York–based makeup artist Rebecca Restrepo shares her tips for applying eyeliner like the experts:

➤ If you're using liquid liner, lightly dust sheer loose powder on your lids first to allow the liquid to adhere better. If you're curling your lashes, do it before eyeliner application.

➤ For a straight line, use a liquid liner, such as Bobbi Brown Gel Eyeliner, or for a softer, smokier look, try Bourjois Twist-Up Liners, which are chalkier and easier to blend.

➤ Rest your elbow on a hard surface to keep your hand from shaking. Start applying from the inner corner of the eye as close to the eyelashes as you can and actually aim for the eyelash in short, connecting strokes until you're all the way across the eye.

➤ If you want to make your eyes look smoky but still want definition, apply a pencil eyeliner and then dab an eye shadow in a similar shade over the top, lightly fanning it out. This will also help the eyeliner stay in place.

ELEGANT EVENING EYES

Make Up For Ever professional makeup artist Careth Whitchurch tells how to achieve a total evening look: "One word: Shimmer. Follow my tips [see "Eyes That Make a Statement," page 68] to determine the best colors for your eyes, and then add a deeper shade all around the lash line and blend for a smoky look. To finalize, use a dark liner and add Make Up For Ever's Star Powder and/or Diamond Powder ($17)."

➤ If your eyeliner smudges, don't be tempted to apply more on top—it's more likely to smudge and won't have a clean finish. Instead, tidy the line with a cotton swab and start again. You can also dip the swab in a nonoily makeup remover, such as Almay, to get a cleaner line without residue.

Blush

Blush is there to add a kiss of color to your cheeks. Just a playful and polite little peck of a kiss, not a big, wet, sloppy, "Come here and give your Auntie Ethel a kiss" kiss; or that face-munching, tongue wrestling, saliva-drenched thing that your first high school boyfriend called a kiss. You'd be surprised how many women get confused.

Powder Blush

HIGH LORAC Cheek Duo and It Kits ($28.50)

Fine department stores or www.sephora.com

Blush can be anticlimactic, yawn-inducing, and even positively traumatic. As a duo or individually, depending on which sun-kissed look you want, LORAC Cheek Duo and It Kits do it all to create natural, healthy sheen with just a "pop" of color that's positively idealized.

HIGH Beauty Addicts Sleek Cheeks ($27)

www.beautyaddicts.com

When you have options, a world of possibilities opens, and that's why we love Beauty Addicts so much. Their cheek duos have both cream and powder blush, and are positively the chicest shades we've discovered.

MEDIUM Cat Cosmetics Whiskers Blush ($14)

www.catcosmetics.com

This is one catalicious blush—the perfect shade of rose pink with a touch of gold looks good on any skin tone, no matter how fair or dark. It's like catnip—you just can't get enough!

LOW L'Oreal Powder Blush ($8.99)

Mass retailers

WAVE YOUR MAGIC WAND

To make eyes pop, celebrity makeup artist Mally Roncal has created the Light Wand, a double-ended wand with one end a soft cap that contains powder, and the other end a soft (but not mushy) pencil in a light shimmer that also looks good on every skin tone. First, use the pencil to gently draw in the inner corner (the sideways V) of your eye. Then, take the other end, a perfect shimmer dust of powder, and soften the "V" by dusting the powder, extending a bit into the inner part of the bridge of the nose. It lightens up the eye area, makes you look as if you've had a great eight hours of sleep, and helps draw attention away from dark circles. You can also use it on your browbone or on your cupid's bow of your lips to make your mouth look poutier ($25; www.qvc.com, item #A57063).

Does selecting the right blush make you fret? Blush gone wrong can be a disaster, but consider this blush form L'Oreal that our league of women testers and experts absolutely swear by. It is so luxurious the price will make you do a double take. The secret to this undeniable blush is that it's jet-milled, which means that it is so fine it glides on effortlessly and edgelessly.

THE AUTHORS' PICK is the Cat Cosmetics Whiskers Blush. It's such perfection on the cheeks that the urge for more goes into overdrive and we are driven by a relentless urge to apply more than we should.

Cream Blush

We are always vexed by cream blush. Seriously, the only people who ever use it seem to be our mothers, and we rarely take beauty or fashion advice from them. But since we honor our mothers, and their wisdom, we thought it wise to include cream blush in this book.

HIGH Beauty Addicts Sleek Cheeks ($27)

www.beautyaddicts.com

Our experts tell us they like the cream because it's a cream-to-powder formula with subtle shimmer that can be used for cheeks, shoulders, or even décolleté. We love it because there's a shade for every skin type and occasion. Also, it glides on effortlessly and adds just the perfect touch of glow, depending on just how flush you're feeling.

HIGH DuWop Blast-from-the-past Blush Therapy Stick ($22)

Fine department stores

The name of this blush is enough of a reason to buy it, and then the breezy application comes in, and you're hooked. Better yet, it's available in six shades, with a hint of aromatherapy so you can sniff your way to happier times as you apply.

MEDIUM Stila Cream Blush ($20)

www.stilacosmetics.com or (877) 737-4672

It melts into your cheeks like buttah and brings out the Barbra Streisand in all of us, but what we really love are the darling shades that complement nearly all skin tones. Apply gently, though; it goes on so smoothly that you can easily overdo it.

LOW Wet 'n' Wild Twist-up Blush Stick ($1.99)

Mass retailers

What really drives us wild about this is the price, but it also comes in a gaggle of shades to make you just ga-ga for hours.

THE AUTHORS' PICK is the DuWop. A bad hair day and last minute outfit change aren't

TOO MUCH BLUSH ALERT!

If you've overdone it and are feeling more circus clown than fashion icon, take a washcloth and run it under water. Wring it out so it's damp, but not wet, and lightly pat your cheeks. This should absorb the extra without the need to rub it off, which can make your cheeks even redder. You want to look exquisite, not embarrassed.

enough to ruin DuWop's hue. We love the shades and can't live without them.

Tints and Stains

What's amazing about tints and stains is the fact that they provide a wash of color that is so subtle others will never be able to quite put their finger on what you're wearing—they will only notice it's fresh, sweet, and a little bit mesmerizing. We love defrosting our cheeks with stains because the look lasts longer than a powder. Here are our experts' favorites, and a few we love, too.

OUTRAGEOUS   pixi Hydrotint Duo ($38)
www.sephora.com

Okay, first of all, the bullet-tipped lip and cheek tint is cool, smooth, and feels great going on. Then there's the moisturizer to brighten and perfect your skin color—it's the ideal duo.

HIGH   LORAC Sheer Wash ($24)
Fine department stores or www.sephora.com

The LORAC gives off just the right wash of color for an irresistible coquettish look that simply says, "I'm trying to be sexy without really trying."

MEDIUM   Benetint Balm ($18)
www.benefitcosmetics.com

The stain that's celebrating twenty years of fame is still the sexiest flush from a bottle. For a ladylike blush, this ruby-tinted cheek and lip stain is innocent enough for school clothes, yet provocative enough for kiss-proof "Honey, I love your lips" evenings by the fire.

LOW   Neutrogena Shimmer Sheers ($8.99)
Mass retailers

The newspaper article simply read: "The night watchman was jumped at gunpoint by what he described as two women in their twenties. Missing items from the drugstore included a box of candy bars, he thinks Twix, a liter of Coca-Cola, and the remaining seven Neutrogena Shimmer Sheers. The watchman did not return our calls for comment, but the drugstore manager said, 'We're really upset that the Neutrogena Shimmer Sheers were taken. It's our most popular product, we can't keep it in stock, and dad-gummit, those two girls took my last seven. Can you imagine?'" Since Neutrogena Shimmer Sheers give you an all-over healthy glow, the perpetrators are known to be armed and fabulous.

THE AUTHORS' PICK is the LORAC Sheer Wash. It gives you a soft glow without being overpowering, as so many tints are. We also love the soft shades that look good on everyone.

IN A CATEGORY OF ITS OWN

We also love the pixi Velvet Rouge ($22; www.sephora.com), but since it's a liquid to powder formation (which is pretty cool in itself), we don't have a category for it. It also works well as a lightweight eye-color base.

THE IT LIST

Michelyn Camen, Hollywood beauty insider (and luxury brand fanatic), gives us her Top Ten Beauty Picks for 2007:

1. Foundation: It's a tie between the **Giorgio Armani Luminous Sheer Foundation** for day and the **Kevyn Aucoin Sensual Skin Enhancer**, mixed with a drop of moisturizer for an airbrushed and not cakey finish.

2. Moisturizer: I've tried everything, including $500-an-ounce moisturizers with caviar, silk, pitera, you name it, but when all is said and done it's about hydration and nonirritating ingredients. The clear winner is **Jo Malone's Ginseng Day Moisturizer**. It's terrific for normal skin and smells heavenly.

3. Brow pencil: **Eliza's Essentials Brunette Chunky Brow Filler** fills in those patches and sparse areas from years of overzealous tweezing. I'm here to tell you, it's natural looking.

4. Eyeshadow: **Kevyn Aucoin Liquid Eye Shading in Peach** brightens my whole face, and you only need a little.

5. Lip pencil: **Giorgio Armani Lip Pencil #7** is the best. I always have a spare hanging around, because the brownish warm shade is a bit deeper than my lips and goes with every lip color I wear.

6. Eyeliner: **YSL Liner Moire in #1** is liquid with a precise brush in a slate, dark gray. I think it's better than black because it doesn't look harsh.

7. **Luckyscent.com** is where I find the most exotic and hard-to-find perfumes and candles. No one else ever has these scents, which truly makes me a beauty insider. Current faves are **Ginestet Sauvignonne** and **Botrytis**, produced by a vineyard in the south of France.

8. Eye cream: I love **Bobbi Brown EXTRA Eye Balm**. It's extremely scary when you open the jar because it looks like congealed Vaseline, but girls, it's unbelievably effective and emollient.

9. Lipstick: I love **Paul and Joe** because the packaging is genius and the product is pigmented but not dry. Great natural colors, too.

10. Eyelash curler: **Cle de Peau** is the clear winner. It's gold-plated and super-luxe looking. It curls my lashes to the max, but here's the problem. You can only buy it in Japan. If I lost it, I would cry.

Bronzing Powders

OUTRAGEOUS **Prescriptives Sunsheen Bronze Trio ($30)**

www.prescriptives.com

You'll sweep from sheer to gold, and the combination of the three shades in one works wonders. Sporting that color boost without four hours in the sun is the creative assist we all need when the heat index is high.

HIGH **Cat Cosmetics Girl on Fire! ($26)**

www.catcosmetics.com

The date you've been hoping for has finally happened, but now it's the witching hour and he still hasn't even gone to first base. Step into the ladies' room, lightly sweep this powder on, and you'll sizzle up so high on the barometer he won't be able to keep his hands off you.

MEDIUM **Physician's Formula Les Botaniques Botanical Bronzer ($12)**

Mass retailers

For those of us who love a healthy glow any time of year, this botanical bronzer warms up the complexion in seconds flat. It contains sunflower extracts and antioxidants so you can brush on the flower power for peaceful skin.

LOW **Bonne Bell Powder Bronze in Golden Tan ($4.49)**

Mass retailers

This is a soft, oil-absorbing powder, so it controls shine and also gives you a radiant, natural-looking tan. At this price, it can't be beat.

THE AUTHORS' PICK is the Cat Cosmetics Girl on Fire! We can't resist all things CAT, it's true, but this truly is our favorite bronzer because it gives you just the right shade of glow, whatever that is.

Lips

Your lips can be your engine of seduction. You want them to be luscious, sexy, sweet, and maybe even a little naughty. You want them to be irresistible magnets of passion. So how do you remind him of the fun of making a family, not the horror of family reunions? Here are some hints.

Long-Lasting Lipstick

OUTRAGEOUS **Sisley Hydrating Long-Lasting Lipstick ($40.00)**

Saks Fifth Avenue, Neiman Marcus, Bergdorf Goodman, and select boutiques

The shape and color of a lipstick is the first impression before you slide it on, and Sisley's new long-lasting lipsticks have the coolest shape we've ever seen. It's a four-sided gem-shaped style in shades so yummy you'll want to suck on

NEED SOME SUGAR?

For super-kissable lips, try Mary Kay Satin Lips Lip Mask and Lip Balm ($9.50, www.marykay.com). First, buff away dry skin with the lip mask, then moisturize with the lip balm.

them like candy. The eye-catching hues stay on your lips all day, and quite frankly, the price works to keep up the image of this continental lipstick.

HIGH   Chanel Ultra Wear Lip Colour ($30)
Fine department stores

A white-hot mama can't sustain the spellbound look if her lip color is fading. Chanel will never let you down. We love this lip color because it lasts and lasts and there's no stinging or side effects from the ingredients. It's the perfect lip pick-me-up.

MEDIUM   Max Factor Lipfinity ($12)
Mass retailers

Max Factor dishes up some serious fantastic paint shades with Lipfinity—and it really does last all day. To remove Lipfinity, use an oil-based makeup remover, baby oil, or petroleum jelly.

LOW   L'Oreal Endless Kissable Lipcolour ($7.99)
Mass retailers

If you're going to push yourself to the limit every day, you want a lip color that meets the challenge. The L'Oreal Kissables stay on edge with you hour to hour, without drying your lips.

THE AUTHORS' PICK: Paula can't resist the Sisley, for the long-lasting effect, and the diamond shape gets her positively flustered. Maureen loves the L'Oreal because it stays from carpool to cocktails and dancing, and isn't drying like most long-wear lipcolor.

Moisturizing Lipstick

HIGH   Estée Lauder Pure Color Lip Vinyl Gloss Stick ($22)
Department stores or www.esteelauder.com

The ultrafeminine look of lipstick gets a flirty finish with this one because it's absolutely the most moisturizing lipstick at this price. It goes on soft and stays this way all day. It's a gorgeous goodie you can't live without.

MEDIUM   Kitten Impossible Lipstick ($16)
www.catcosmetics.com

Cat gets the award, hands down, for best packaging. This lipstick comes so cleverly designed with a mirror that folds up when you pop the top off. If that weren't enough, Cat has designed

RED RULES

Did you ever wonder why someone else looks better in red lipstick than you? It's probably because you're not selecting the right red for your skin tone. Everyone wants that 50s Hollywood glamour, the velvety-textured red pouts made famous by the likes of Rita Hayworth, but getting that look is a bit trickier than just slapping on color. Gordon Elliott, the celebrity makeup artist for MAC Cosmetics, offers the following tips on finding the right red for you. "Blue-based reds and dark wine are usually best on mid-toned olive and darker skins, while clear to yellow based or orange reds are best suited to paler complexions. For someone with a lot of red in their skin, opt for a red that is muted with a bit more terra-cotta or plum. Also, use a brush to apply red lipstick for a perfect pout."

shades that look great on everyone, and they're velvety soft. We love you, Cat!

LOW Maybelline New York Moisture Extreme Lipstick ($7)

Mass retailers

It's a leap of faith when you purchase a lipstick that claims to last all day and moisturize. This is not only a long-wearing lipstick, but the colors stay true all day with a light, creamy formulation that also provides instant moisture.

THE AUTHORS' PICK for Paula is the Estee Lauder because it feels softer and smoother than any lipstick she's ever tried. The pick for Maureen is the Maybelline New York Moisture Extreme because, as she says, "I just can't pin down a smoother lipstick at a price that leaves me feeling positively jazzy."

Lip Tints

For that succulent just-bitten look, you can't beat the right lip tint. Just like tints and stains for the cheeks, lip tints provide a perfect wash of color to perfect your pretty pout. We are amazed that science has finally allowed the tint to emerge. They come in many applications: with a brush, with a felt tip like a marker, in a lipstick, or even as a balm. We like to wear them alone with gloss layered over on them, and our professionals tell us that lip tints are also a good base color for lipsticks and tinted glosses. Whatever your lip tint fantasy, we have several options for you here.

HIGH pixi Lip Blush ($20)

www.pixibeauty.com

Just because you're not a little girl any more doesn't mean you can't play with markers. It's like coloring your face with a jumbo felt-tip marker in six sexy shades that tint your lips naturally and are water-resistant, too. They'll say, "She's very sweet, isn't she?" as they fuss over those pixi lips.

MEDIUM Benetint Lip Balm ($18)

www.benefitcosmetics.com

Every time we find another wonderful Benefit product we feel as if we've been thrown yet another curveball. Their products always pack a punch that we can't see coming. The Benefit Benetint Balm is the envy of all others because it consistently works not only for lips but for cheeks as well. Referring back to Beauty Buyble Commandment #8 (page x), please note that we do not advocate lipstick as rouge. This is a tint, not a lipstick so get your facts straight before you send us letters of complaint.

MEDIUM MAC Tint Toons ($14)

www.maccosmetics.com

LIP TO HAIR TIP

If flyaway hairs are in your way and you don't have hair spray on hand, take small amount of clear lip gloss and rub gently through the tips of your fingers. Then lightly brush your fingers over the hairs you want to tame for instant control.

We're spellbound. The MAC shades range from Popsicle purples to pop star pinks and everything in between. They never dry the lips, as so many tints do, and the irresistible shades can literally change your overall skin tone from flat to fantastic. And yes, we know it's a bit pricey, but it's worth it.

LOW **Too Faced Bunny Balm ($11)**
www.sephora.com

Too Faced Bunny Balm is a zero-calorie lip balm packed with guava, pineapple, ginger, and grapefruit essential oils, which means it smells like a delicious exotic tropical fruit salad and keeps your lips soft, supple, and just as tasty. It's a calorie-free, carb-free lip diet that you can take to the office or to bed for a sweet treat.

THE AUTHORS' PICK is a split lip. Paula loves the MAC Tint Toons because what's more fun than a lip tint with a cartoon character endorsement? Maureen loves the Too Faced Bunny Balm because it's satiny smooth and oh-so-affordable.

Clear Gloss

Sometimes we just want a shiny hiney. So we rub a mixture of lip gloss, Magic Shell, and carnauba wax on our bottoms and then buff them liberally with a portable electric router with chamois attachment. Oh, wait, we're talking about lips here. Never mind. Sometimes we just want a touch of gloss for some big-time shine. Since the use of industrial varnishes and shellacs can be stunning but painful and highly toxic, the *Beauty Buyble* suggests you try a clear gloss to give your lips that patent leather shine.

HIGH **CITY Cosmetics CITY Lips ($29)**
Fine department stores

There's a special ingredient in this gloss called Celadrol that enhances collagen production to increase lip volume and reduce lip lines. The result is full, soft, pouty lips while you gloss.

MEDIUM **Benefit's The Gloss ($14)**
www.benefitcosmetics.com

Did we tell you that we really like Benefit? The Gloss is another great product in their lineup; it's not ooey-gooey and it doesn't wear off minutes after you apply it.

MEDIUM **MAC Lipglass ($11) (also available with tint for $13.50)**
www.maccosmetics.com

MAC Lipglass goes on thick, giving your lips the ultimate glassy look, with extreme shine and moisturization that lasts for hours. MAC LipGlass

LIP LOLLIES

Chupa Chup has teamed up with Lotta Luv to make a delicious lip gloss and a bevy of other beauty bites that will have your mouth watering with anticipation. We're positively giddy that they decided to team up with The Beauty Buyble *and create a flavor just for us: Watermelon. We'd love to know what you think of the new flavor!*

junkies include Chloe Sevigny, Linda Evangelista, Missy Elliot, and Christina Aguilera.

LOW   Maybelline Lip Polish ($5.49)

Mass retailers

The gel-based formula delivers bombshell shine at a fraction of the cost of the other clear glosses.

THE AUTHORS' PICK is the MAC. It's super clear and shiny and never gives your lips that gummy feeling as it dries. It keeps lips super-soft and poufy, and we love that.

Gloss with Tint or Shimmer

HIGH   Versace Lights on Lips ($22)

www.buycosmetics.com or
www.strawberrynet.com

It's a shocking shine, but this lip gloss is without question the most sparkling ever created. The formulation includes special polymer shining agents with glitter and gelatinizing substances. We admit that this gloss is a tad on the gooey side, but oh, it's worth it because it stays on for hours. We are addicted and really bummed because you can no longer buy this in the United States (Versace discontinued their U.S. beauty distribution), and the only way we could find it is at the websites above.

MEDIUM   Lipmints ($14)

www.lip-mints.com

Each lip gloss is infused with spearmint flavor to add a surprising zing of fresh mint when a toothbrush and toothpaste aren't handy. It's also a very smooth, nonsticky formulation that glides on easily. There are six Lipmints: Mint Lust, Mint Vogue, Mint Love, Mint Naked, Mint Sweetheart, and Mint Pout.

LOW   Sally Hansen Diamond Lip Treatment ($4.95)

Mass retailers

Stops dry lips with generous amounts of shea butter and puts out some serious 3-D shine with unbelievably bright, eye-catching colors.

LOW   N.Y.C. Pencil & Pout ($3.99)

Mass retailers

This is a true double-duty product with a smooth lip pencil on one end and a rich shiny gloss on the other. The shades are divine.

e.l.f.   Hypershine Gloss ($1)

Mass retailers

The idea that we can find a beauty product so superior at an unreal price is still alien to us, but the fact is that the e.l.f. Hypershine Gloss is super cheap and goes on as wet and slick as these others. Why wouldn't you use it?

GOOD GOLLIE MS. GOLDIE!

The Goldie Lip Gloss reigns supreme in its own category because it's the perfect formula; not sticky and not slippery. We love all the shades: Sherry Cherry, Baby, Naked, Whip It, Brownie, Doll, Cream, Leslie, Snowfox, Velveteen, Pomme, Dressed, Blossom, April, Nylon, and Clean Sheets. $14, Bath & Body Works flagship stores.

THE AUTHORS' PICK is the e.l.f Hypershine Gloss for Maureen because at this price she just can't change her view, and the Versace Lights on Lips for Paula. It's really frustrating that this product isn't readily available, but it's worth the extra effort to find it.

Lip Plumpers

They can sting and they're extreme, but if you want to plump those lips in a hurry for Mr. Right Now, you need a lip plumper. Some good news: they don't *have* to sting to work, there are a few alternatives in our pick of the best, and we have quite a few here, so you can't lose. Our only challenge in this category, however, was finding anything truly affordable. Seems big lips come with a rather plump price tag, too!

HIGH Freeze 24/7 Plump Lips ($40)

Henri Bendel, Sephora, Louis Boston, Zitomers, Stanley Korshak Greenhouse Spa, other fine stores, or www.freeze247.com

It's clear, nonsticky, and puffs your lips like freshly plumped pillows. The proprietary blend of ingredients is mostly a mystery, much like Watergate but without Deep Throat, and includes niacin, retinol, and white orchid.

HIGH LipFusion Lip Pump ($36)

Sephora stores or www.sephora.com

While many facial products list collagen as a key ingredient, in actuality, the collagen molecule is too large to penetrate the skin. LipFusion's patented technology dehydrates the collagen molecule into tiny microspheres that can infiltrate the lip tissue and then search for the body's natural water to rehydrate up to fifty times their size, creating a beautiful full-on pout. This microinjected collagen lip plump works without injection and gives your lips the ultimate bee-stung appearance without the pain and agony of sitting in a doctor's office. It takes about two minutes for results, but plumpness lasts for up to forty-eight hours.

HIGH The Hollywood Prescription Two-Step Lip Treatment ($29)

www.hollywoodrx.com

This system begins with the Exfoliant, which you use two or three times a week to slough off dead skin on your lips to keep them smooth. Then, apply step two, the Lip Serum. This clear gel uses proprietary ingredients to permanently plump lips (with continued use).

HIGH Philosophy Big Mouth ($25)

www.philosophy.com

Naturalists will love Philosophy Big Mouth because there's no microinjection or overly pumped chemicals to big-up your lips. Instead, it's a lip primer, which enhances the appearance of natu-

LIP NIBBLERS

We are crazy over Cat Cosmetics Lip Nibblers ($16, www.catcosmetics.com). They're a tinted gloss and lip hydrator and softener in one. We apply the nibblers at bedtime for some under the sheets glamour while fortifying our lips, and during the day to add just a touch of tempting texture or sparkling shimmer.

ral color and shape of lips for the bee-stung look without the sting. Big Mouth comes in Pink or Nude.

THE AUTHORS' PICK is the Freeze 24/7, hands down. There's an intense rush of plumping action for a few minutes, but don't worry, it's sooooo worth it.

PARIS HILTON'S BEAUTY SECRETS

Paris Hilton shared her deepest, darkest, and most coveted beauty secrets with us:

➤ Lips: The most important feature on your face is your lips. Change your lipstick color often and make sure your lips are always moist and healthy. Nothing works better than using The Hollywood Prescription ($29; www.hollywoodrx.com) every day to achieve beautiful, perfect-looking lips.

➤ Cleansing: Always wash off your makeup before going to sleep. If you don't, your skin will not be able to breathe properly, and this can cause blemishes. It takes only a couple of minutes. After a hard day of work or a night on the town, I always make sure to remove my makeup.

➤ Eye cream: It's never too early or too late to start using eye cream. The sensitive skin around eyes needs extra protection to help prevent fine lines, wrinkles, and sagging. It will also make you look more refreshed during the day.

➤ Sunblock: Always wear SPF of at least 15 during the day. The sun has harmful rays that can cause premature aging and cancer. The Los Angeles sun is always shining, so I make sure not to leave the house without it on. Even if you don't live in Hollywood, you should always apply SPF.

➤ Exfoliation: It's important to exfoliate your face twice a week. This removes dead skin cells that can build up and clog pores. Be sure to use a gentle exfoliant, however, so as not to irritate skin. I like to follow this with a lightweight moisturizer.

➤ Hair: Change your look and hairstyle often. It keeps you interesting and makes you stand out.

➤ Water: Drink plenty of water all day long. Your skin needs water to stay hydrated, and when skin is hydrated it produces a natural, healthy glow. It also flushes unwanted toxins out of your body. I drink at least six bottles of water a day to keep my skin looking beautiful.

A POUT TO COVET

Make Up For Ever professional makeup artist Careth Whitchurch gives the following tips on how to get fuller-looking lips: "Choose a lip liner one shade darker than your lips/lipstick and use it to shade rather than just to line. Darken corners and bring slightly lower than the natural lip. After applying lipstick, highlight the center of the lip, top and bottom, with a lighter gloss."

Lip Moisturizers / Balms

We can't live without lip moisturizers and lip balms—they're minature life preservers for the lips. A good lip moisturizer and you're worry-free from dry lips for a lifetime, they're that important. We all know what happens when our lips get overly dry; cracking, flaking, and sometimes bleeding. No, ladies, we cannot have this, so trust us when we say, "Do not go out without a good lip moisturizer or balm in your bag," and take our advice on the top picks from our beauty experts.

HIGH Prada Shielding Balm with SPF 15 ($38 for 8, ½-ounce single-doses in individually sealed packages)

Neiman Marcus, Barneys New York, select Saks Fifth Avenue stores, select Prada stores, or www.neimanmarcus.com

At this price you may purchase it kicking and screaming all the way, but we swear by this balm. This is a thick, highly emollient balm, loaded with shea butter. Better yet, it contains sunscreen filters to soften the lips but also protect them from UVA and UVB rays. Celebrities who don't leave home without it include Madonna, Uma Thurman, Renee Zellweger, and Brad Pitt.

LOW Burt's Bees Lip Shimmers ($3.50)
www.burtsbees.com

A kiss of color has been added to Burt's Bees' World's Best Lip Balm so you can protect and moisturize while showing off just a touch of luminescent color. Available in seven different shades.

YOUR DAILY DQ

We all scream for ice cream, and Lotta Luv somehow managed to get the rights to create **Lotta Luv's Dairy Queen Balms** to satisfy your sweet tooth and soften your lips. All eight balms are good enough to eat. Whatever you're craving, there is a flavor for you:

➤ DQ Strawberry Sundae Lip Balm

➤ DQ Chocolate Sundae Lip Balm

➤ DQ Vanilla Sundae Lip Balm

➤ DQ Chocolate Dipped Cone Lip Balm

➤ DQ Vanilla Dipped Cone Lip Balm

➤ DQ Strawberry Dipped Cone Lip Balm

➤ DQ Vanilla Ice Cream Lip Gloss

➤ DQ Butterscotch Ice Cream Lip Gloss

It's ice cream, minus the guilt. What could be better, and at $3 to $5, we couldn't resist getting each of them. Available through www.lottaluv.com.

LOW   Natural Ice ($.97)
Kmart and Wal-Mart

At 97 cents you'll be as impressed with the price as with the results. It's amazing we didn't know about it sooner! If the $38 price tag of the Prada Shielding Balm is just too much for your budget, we highly recommend Natural Ice.

THE AUTHORS' PICK is the Prada Shielding Balm. It is clearly the best lip moisturizer on the market, bar none, and justifies its cost.

Lip Liners

When you were a little girl (or boy—we don't discriminate here at the *Beauty Buyble*), didn't you always wish for a magic wand that you could wave and you'd look magnificent? Well, this is real life honey, and we've all learned that the length and power of most wands are greatly *greatly* exaggerated. Still, we have a little spark of magic for you in the form of lip liners. These wands will give you full, pouty lips, sleek elegant lips, or just simply clean lines to keep your lipstick from bleeding. Just a deft wave and presto—an instantly fabulous kisser!

HIGH   Chanel Le Crayon Lèvres Precision Lip Definer ($26.50)
Fine department stores

The Chanel Lip Definer is a time-tested product that stands up to even the most discriminating lips. We love this liner because it never feels dry going on, and Chanel always delivers the boldest, most incredible shades.

MEDIUM   DuWop Reverse Lip Liner ($19)
Department stores

A good lip liner should help prevent your lipstick from feathering and bleeding, and this one does the job. We love it because you don't get those harsh lines seen with most lip liners and the unique ingredient Kambuchka—derived from wild mushrooms from Tibet—is known to help plump and fill the lips where volume is needed. Oh, it also comes with a custom sharpener.

LOW   N.Y.C. Waterproof Lipliner Pencil ($3.99)
Mass retailers

If you're devoted to lip rituals, you're probably going through a lot of lip liner. The N.Y.C lip liner delivers perfection at a price you won't have to suffer.

THE AUTHORS' PICK is the Chanel. While the lip-lining trend comes and goes, we stick with Chanel because it's nearly impossible to mess up and the shades are divine.

Teeth Whitening

Earth tones are wonderful for cosmetics. Tans and yellows can make a woman look elegant, while black can add a dramatic flair. However, tan, yellow, and black don't work so well when it comes to teeth. Ladies, the only blacks and tans that should be near your lips are the ones the boys will line up to buy for you at the bar when you flash that winning white smile of yours.

Shiny, white, sinless teeth give you that movie star impression when you break a smile. Dr. Michael Ghalili, an associate professor and director of the International General Dentistry Program at New York University College of Dentistry in New York City, answered our most pressing questions about teeth whitening (and he would know; he tends to some of the most important celebrity choppers on the red carpet).

Why is teeth whitening so popular?

I think that people are more conscious about their appearance in general and their teeth in particular than they have been in the past. Also, the producers of whitening products have done an excellent job of marketing.

How does it work?

There are several types of tooth whitening products:

➤ In-office procedures: a whitening gel is applied to the teeth, and then the patient is placed under a special light, often confused with a laser, for about one hour. The light activates and accelerates the whitening effect of the gel. It is very important to protect the gums and skin around the mouth since the gel and light can be extremely irritating to these areas. When done by a properly trained dentist, it is a very safe and effective procedure. Patients will usually need to repeat the procedure once per year.

➤ Take-home trays: the dentist makes a mold of the teeth and creates a clear plastic tray that fits snugly over the patient's teeth. The patient applies the whitening gel inside the tray and then places the tray over the teeth. Depending on the manufacturer, the tray should be worn for one to eight hours per day for five to ten days. The trays can also be used as an adjunct treatment after an in-office whitening procedure. This ensures the maximum result. The at-home treatment can be repeated every three to four months as necessary to maintain the whitening effect.

➤ Whitening strips: these are mass-produced strips with whitening material impregnated directly onto the strip. The patient simply applies the strip over the teeth for one hour to over night, depending on the product. There are higher concentration strips available in dental offices and lower concentration strips available over the counter.

What over-the-counter products do you recommend?

I recommend Crest White Strips. They are safe, relatively effective, and easy to use. However it's a fairly time-consuming process, due to their low concentrations of whitening gel.

Makeup Removers

The days of using soap and water to remove makeup are decades behind us, but it's still a hassle trying to figure out which makeup removers really work. They're either too runny or too thick, or they sting your eyes. Stop the frenzy—here are some makeup removers that will leave you squeaky clean without the negative side effects.

MEDIUM Kiehl's Supremely Gentle Eye Makeup Remover ($15.50)

www.kiehls.com

Kiehl's makeup remover has long been a favorite among makeup artists nationwide. It removes thoroughly and without leaving the skin feeling greasy.

MEDIUM Mustela PhysiObébé No-Rinse Cleansing Fluid ($13.50)

Sephora or www.mustelausa.com

Mustela PhysiObébé is a one-step no-rinse cleanser for the face that is so gentle it's used by mothers everywhere to clean their babies. Since it doesn't contain soap and is safe for eyes, moms also love this for taking off their eye makeup. Simply pump a small amount on a cotton ball and gently remove makeup.

LOW Maybelline Expert Eyes 100% Oil Free Make-Up Remover ($4.65)

Mass retailers

We have a penchant for anything that works and doesn't break the bank. But when it really works, doesn't irritate your eyes, and takes that makeup off swiftly without residue, well then we have to tell you that this makeup remover is the perfect strategy to wipe away the day.

THE AUTHORS' PICK is the Mustela because it's extremely gentle, won't irritate the skin, and smells fresh and heavenly.

MUSTELA MOMENT

Mustela products have been used by mothers for more than fifty years and have become moms' most coveted product on baby's beauty shelf. Here are just a few nifty everyday uses for Mustela products:

➤ Mustela Dermo-Cleansing is a soap-free cleanser for scalp and body of newborns and babies. Moms love it for shaving their legs. ($16)

➤ Mustela Hydra-Stick with Cold Cream protects sensitive and overexposed areas (lips, cheeks) and ensures long-lasting protection. It is perfect as a lip balm, alone, or under lipstick, and great to stick in the pocket of your ski parka so you can moisturize on the slopes! ($8) Men love it, too, and we like to say it gives you "kissable" lips.

➤ Mustela Musti Eau de Soin is an alcohol-free scent for babies and children that blends floral and fruit tones for a light, fresh scent. It's also perfect for any adult, particularly if you are sensitive to alcohol-based perfumes. ($27.50) Many expectant moms also use Musti, as they often cannot tolerate their normal heavier perfume.

For additional information visit www.mustelausa.com. To purchase Mustela products, visit a Sephora store or go to www.sephora.com.

Facial Cleansers

A critical part of your beauty regimen is your facial cleanser. Not only does it remove your makeup, but it also removes the dirt and grime of living, leaving your face clean and refreshed and your pores clear. Think of yourself as a great artist; a good facial cleanser assures that you have a fresh and clean canvas to work with every day.

Foaming Cleansers

Most of us are used to some foam when we cleanse, and we've come to equate the foaming experience with clean. The truth is that we don't actually need foam to clean, but for traditionalists here are some elegant foaming cleansers that won't irritate your skin.

HIGH Jurlique Foaming Facial Cleanser ($52)

www.jurlique.com

We understand why Jurlique has such a loyal cult following; there's something truly elegant about this facial wash, from the floral essences aroma to the rich lather. After the experience your skin feels squeaky clean and fresh.

MEDIUM DHC Mild Soap ($14)

www.dhccare.com

Tired of being upstaged by beauty insiders know which facial soaps work best? Take DHC Mild Soap is great for all skin types leaves your skin refreshingly clean without tight, itchy feeling. We love this clear simple bar and the three-piece set includes a soap carrying case for those who travel.

MEDIUM CeraVe Hydrating Cleanser ($11.40)

Drugstores

No matter how you slice it, combining a great facial wash with hydration is a challenge, but we love the CeraVe because it was developed by dermatologists, is soap-free and fragrance-free, and works well on nearly all skin types.

LOW N.Y.C. Foaming Facial Cleanser ($4.99)

Drugstores

Rumors about facial cleansers never end. This one's too drying, this one's too oily—good grief! The N.Y.C. cleanser is a well-kept secret; it's gentle and light and never leaves the skin feeling dry. It also seems to work well with nearly all skin types.

OFF IN A FLASH

DHC Make-off Sheets are stand-alones in the makeup remover sheets category. For $6 you get fifty sheets made of 100 percent cotton, so it's gentle on your skin. Aloe, chamomile, ginseng, and citric acid remove dirt and makeup while depositing moisture, and the flip-top box is adorable and easy to take on the road or to the gym.

THE AUTHORS' PICK is the N.Y.C. Foaming Facial Cleanser because it lathers and moisturizes with the same intensity, and never feels drying to the skin.

Nonfoaming Cleansers

The secret to nonfoaming cleansers is no sodium laureth sulfate, the same ingredient that foams shampoo. The fact is that you don't need all that foam to clean your face. For those seeking a purer and less chemical-filled way to clean, here are some great foam-free facial cleansers.

HIGH Environ Interactive Cleansing Cream ($30)

(212) 750-7100

You'll have to go a little out of the way for this one because Environ skin care products must be purchased through a medical office. Dr. Philip Miller, a plastic surgeon in New York City, introduced us to the line, and we fell in love with the Environ Interactive Cleansing Cream because it is so gentle and works well on all skin types.

HIGH DHC Deep Cleansing Oil ($24)

www.dhccare.com

This is a truly amazing cleanser that removes everything, even waterproof mascara, and you don't even need to add water until you're ready to rinse it off. The fruit oils and olive oils leave your skin positively plush!

MEDIUM Cetaphil Gentle Skin Cleanser ($11.50)

Mass retailers

Cris Osborn, Ph.D., medical director of Galderma Laboratories, makers of Cetaphil, says: "It's the undeniable matriarch of skin cleansers, the leader upon which so many brands have been patterned. It offers anyone of any age unsurpassed gentleness, safety, and efficacy. She may be over fifty, but she still keeps skin looking young and radiant. Recommended by thousands of dermatologists worldwide, Cetaphil Gentle Skin Cleanser for Normal to Dry Skin and Cetaphil Daily Facial Cleanser for Normal to Oily Skin are free of soap, fragrance, and common irritants, making them ideal for use on sensitive skin."

SECRET FROM THE FAR EAST

We just discovered Nufolia, a new hypoallergenic cleansing system and tightly held beautification secret from Tibet. The face and body mitts are designed for men and women and are created with microfibers from Japan. The fibers have the ability to remove makeup and residue, exfoliate the dead skin cells gently, and deeply cleanse the pores without causing irritation or damage to the skin that we can get from conventional facecloths. The Nufolia soap bar is handmade by cold processing, which preserves the valuable benefits of the sea buckthorn pulp and seed oil (regenerating skin cells, promoting natural antiaging benefits, and calming rosacea). There are no chemicals and no unnatural preservatives. Find the product line at www.nufolia.com; $10 for soap bar, $14 for deluxe soap bar.

LOW **Purpose Gentle Cleansing Wash ($6)**

Mass retailers

There is nothing hush-hush about the fact that this cleansing wash is used by a long list of Hollywood A-listers and dermatologists, and we find it amazing that like Cetaphil it has stood the test of time. It gently cleans and makes the most of your beautiful skin.

THE AUTHORS' PICK for Paula is the Cetaphil. This is truly the star facial cleanser bar none and works on nearly all skin types. It can't be beat in any price range. Maureen's pick is the Environ. She says "I love the way it de-junks my face while leaving it soft and fresh feeling."

FACE YOUR SINS

David Tippe, an endermologist and owner and founder of the Anti-Aging Clinic in Lauderhill, Florida, cites the following as the top skin commandments:

➤ Don't squeeze or pick pimples because the chemicals contained in a pimple are toxic. You can spread those chemicals to other areas of your skin, causing additional breakouts.

➤ Don't apply makeup to an unwashed face. The old products, dirt, and grime are in your pores, and you must remove this buildup before you reapply.

➤ Don't overcleanse your skin, because this strips away the acid mantle, your first line of defense against the elements.

➤ Don't use comedogenic (pore-clogging) products, which include some perfumes and coloring used in many types of makeup. Look for noncomedogenic labels.

➤ Don't sleep in your makeup because this allows the toxins to build up on the face overnight, which will further irritate and disturb your skin. The pores need to be cleaned at least twice a day (morning and evening).

➤ Don't smoke. Smoke creates billions of free radicals, which makes it hard for your skin to repair the damage done in everyday life.

➤ Don't skip sun protection. Most sunscreens block only the UVB rays, the ones that burn the skin and cause pain. But UVA rays are the ones that age the skin and cause cancer, so if you don't use your full-spectrum sunblock to block the UVB and UVA rays, you're purposefully aging your skin.

➤ Don't ignore product instructions. Labels tell you how to use the product to get the maximum performance.

WHIP IT UP

Another find we can't help raving about is the BORBA Fiber-Knit facial cleansers in Replenishing for dry, sensitive, or dehydrated skin; Age Defying for aging skin, fine lines, and wrinkles; and Clarifying for oily skin, breakouts, and pore cleansing. The whipped cleansers are all $3 and contain actual silk fibers to keep skin soft and smooth ($18 and up; www.borba.net)

SKIN CLARITY

The Clarisonic Skin Care Brush ($195) is a deep-cleaning brush with sonic technology that can be used on all skin types to work deep within the skin and pores to loosen dirt and oil. Imagine our delight when we noticed the years just fading away after using this brush!

➤ Don't apply fading or whitening products all over the face—only put them where you need them. Particular whitening products are designed to work not only on the surface of the skin but down below the surface, so if you whiten all over the face, some areas will become too light, resulting in a checkerboard appearance. Not very attractive!

➤ Don't use unsanitary tools and sponges or unclean hands to remove makeup. For example, if you dip your finger in a jar of eye cream, you're placing bacteria from your finger into the jar, and very quickly you could have a product rendered useless from the bacteria. This can even cause more breakouts on your face. Instead, use a plastic spatula to get your product out and then clean the spatula in alcohol before each use. The same applies to sponges—toss them out after each use.

➤ Wash your pillowcases with a low-pH antibacterial soap. This will kill the bacteria that collect from your face and hair, but not leave a high-pH residue that will damage your face's acid mantle.

Under-Eye Treatments

For most short-term eye emergencies, an under-eye concealer will usually do the trick to hide dark circles and eye puffiness. However, some of us need to bring out the heavy artillery to deal with more chronic problems and keep our eyes the center of attention in a positive way. We just have to ask why all the best under-eye treatments are on the pricy side. Isn't there anyone out there making a cheap eye miracle treatment?

OUTRAGEOUS **BORBA Fiber-Knit Orbital Eye Rejuvenator ($65)**
www.borba.net

A REFINED GLOW

For instant skin gratification, try the Mary Kay TimeWise Microdermabrasion set ($55, www.marykay.com). Step 1 contains microfine crystals in a lush exfoliating cream to polish your skin and remove the dull, dry skin on the surface. Step 2 is a nourishing serum that is absorbed instantly to smooth and soothe the skin. The afterglow is transforming!

This dense concoction is as expensive as it is thick, but here's the good news. You only need to dab a small amount to feel and see the effects of this wonder cream. A collagen peptide increases the rate of elastin synthesis, which helps to reduce fine lines, wrinkles, and crow's feet. You should also notice those dark circles diminishing and a decrease in puffiness under the eyes. At least your eyes will be toned!

OUTRAGEOUS Naturpathica Evening Primrose Replenishing Eye Cream ($42)
Leading spas and resorts, 1 (800) 669-7618, or www.naturopathica.com

Most eye creams contain waxes to moisturize, which actually increase puffiness around the eyes. Naturpathica uses a waxless formula, blended with rich evening primrose and borage seed, which are high in anti-oxidants and will hydrate and smooth delicate eye tissue. Essential fatty acids support collagen synthesis to smooth out fine lines and wrinkles around eyes. We can't afford this either. In fact, we can't afford anything by Naturpathica, but we'll tell you that the products are very good despite the ticket price.

MEDIUM Olay Regenerist Eye Lifting Serum ($19)
Mass retailers

If you wake up with a beauty bummer, this is the product to reach for. This eye lifting serum is great for helping to diminish dark circles and de-puff overstressed eyes in a jiffy.

MEDIUM Olay Total Effects Eye Transforming Cream ($19)
Mass retailers

Improves dullness for a radiant glow, evens skin tone, lessens the appearance of dark circles, visibly reduces the look of fine lines and wrinkles, intensively hydrates dry skin, softens uneven texture, minimizes puffiness . . . blah, blah, blah, blah, blah . . . we just love it, okay? Isn't that enough?

MEDIUM NIVEA Q10 Advanced Wrinkle Reduce Eye Crème with SPF 4 ($10.99)
Mass retailers

This creamy blend contains an energy complex with coenzyme Q10 and creatine that reduces wrinkles and helps prevent new ones. Apply a dab of the crème to the outer part of the eye. You can wear it alone or under makeup.

LOW Preparation H Cooling Gel ($12)
Mass retailers

It's typically used for . . . ahem . . . hemorrhoids, but fashion models and Hollywood A-listers have

CONCENTRATION IS KEY

What's loaded with humectants and brightens tired eyes with horse chestnut, ginseng, rosemary, and vitamin E? Still not sure? Okay, we'll tell you.

DHC Concentrated Eye Cream ($29) www.dhccare.com
It wards off wrinkling while conditioning your vulnerable under-eye area skin to become softer. Now that's a bright eye-dea!

known about this secret remedy for under-eye puffiness for years. Use it when you're recovering from a serious night out and your bags are big enough to fill with your groceries.

THE AUTHORS' PICK is the NIVEA because it yields big results at a small price.

Face Scrubs/ Exfoliators

OUTRAGEOUS Canyon Ranch Daily Facial Scrub ($80.00)
www.canyonranch.com

Would anyone really want to pay $80 for a facial scrub? Not really—that is, until you've tried this one. The base is a creamy blend with fine granules that polish the skin gently, without leaving your skin feeling raw.

HIGH Benefit "HONEY . . . snap out of it!" ($23)
www.benefitcosmetics.com

From the eye-catching titles for beauty products to the clever designs, we are unabashedly in love with the Benefit brand (despite the fact that they didn't provide samples for the book and we all know they must be crazy for that poor marketing

decision!). This scrub looks and smells as good as it sounds and ever-so-gently exfoliates your skin to a nice dewy glow.

MEDIUM DHC Facial Scrub ($15)
www.dhccare.com

The apricot seed granules in this scrub are finely milled and rounded for better buffing and the allantoin soothes the skin. Whatever you think of facial scrubs, there's no denying the powerful presence of this one since it's one of our experts' top picks.

LOW Clean & Clear Blackhead Clearing Scrub ($5)
Mass retailers

Your company is requested at the party of the season. You've found just the right little black dress, but what about those blackheads you've been meaning to tackle? You can't very well show up without a fresh face, so you hop in your new red convertible and dash to the drugstore for some Clean & Clear Blackhead Clearing Scrub. Next day, all clear. Now you're sure to dazzle the party circuit from head to toe.

THE AUTHORS' PICK is the Canyon Ranch, hands down. It's true, few can afford it, but we urge you to save your pennies and get some. This scrub is so gentle, yet effective, and it didn't irritate our skin or turn it pink from the scrubbing.

BRIGHT EYES

Medium: DHC Eye Bright ($20, www.dhccare.com) stimulates worn-looking eyes with caffeine and licorice, and soothes with cucumber and other moisture-magnet ingredients. We love the way it reduces puffiness and brightens dark circles.

Toners

A toner is a curious thing. What exactly it does has always been a mystery to most women, but here's the skinny: it's meant to refresh and rejuvenate the skin whenever you feel you need it. It cleans, smooths, acts as an anti-inflamatory, and helps minimize pores while also preventing breakouts. We love it because it gives your skin a boost, good tone, and a healthy glow.

HIGH Fresh Soy Face Cleanser ($35)
www.fresh.com

If you thought you've been there and done that, this is the ultimate salad for the face. Soy promotes moisture retention and firmness, and cucumber extract and rose water refresh and tone. It cleanses the skin, removes makeup quickly without irritation, conditions the eyelashes, and tones the skin.

MEDIUM Prescriptives Immediate Matte ($18.50)
Department stores

A toner by any other name would be snake oil. Prescriptives has truly hit the mark with their Immediate Matte; it cleans pores, tightens skin, and helps even skin tone by getting the shine out. Let's face it—a great pair of butt-fitting jeans and perfect skin make you an irresistible commodity.

LOW L'Oreal Plenitude HydraFresh Toner ($5.49)
Mass retailers

This is an alcohol-free toner, which means it won't dry out your skin and the vitamin B helps prevent moisture loss. It's quite a sophisticated product for the price.

THE AUTHORS' PICK is the L'Oreal. We love the fresh scent and way it makes our skin feel tight and perfectly toned without the harshness of alcohol, while also diminishing the size of our pores.

MARATHON MOISTURE

Put your moisturizer on steroids with DHC Mild Lotion ($28, www.dhccare.com). It's a revitalizing tonic that helps your moisturizer go the extra mile to keep your skin fresh and hydrated. It's also alcohol-free and contains cucumber juice that soothes the skin.

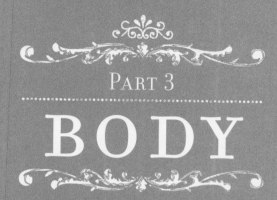

PART 3

BODY

As most legal scholars know, "Habeus Corpus" is an old Roman pick-up line meaning, "You have the body." Some things never change. While a pretty face is an eye-catching hood ornament, it is the chassis that really gets all fine car enthusiasts revved up. With the products we recommend here, your body will scream, "Mercedes" or "Maserati," and not "Yugo."

Please note that we are using the car analogy because it is the number two thing on most men's minds and we just couldn't come up with a good and printable body analogy for the number one thing on most men's minds. We could have gone with number three and said the face was like "toppings," and the body was the "crust," but editorially, we decided that the term "crust" to describe any *Beauty Buyble* girl's body was totally inappropriate and "stuffed crust" was just beyond the pale, no matter how attractive the image is to men.

Sun Protection

Sunscreen

Ever had a friend who turned out to really be your worst enemy? She seemed warm and kind, but did all kinds of harm behind your back. Well, you have one of those right now, and its name is the sun. Yes, the sun does a lot of good things for you, but also gives you wrinkles, dry skin, and even melanomas if you are overexposed. Like most friends, you still need to be careful, and a little SPF goes a long way. A lot of SPF is even better. Forewarned is forearmed.

OUTRAGEOUS Jurlique Herbal Sun Lotion SPF 30+ ($63)
www.jurlique.com

It has an outrageous price, but also an outrageous list of celebrity fans. And for good reason; there are few sunscreens with an SPF this high that go on so sheer and light you can't feel it on the skin. Better yet, it smells great.

HIGH Bliss Oil-Free Sunban Lotion SPF 20 ($25)
Bliss spa locations or www.blissworld.com

To prevent sun rays that cause searing, sizzling, spotting, or sagging, simply swipe on this sumptuous sunban to saturate your sexy self with something that will keep it safe and sumptuous. Sound simple?

MEDIUM Blue Lizard Australian Skincream Lotion ($10.99–$16.99)
Drugstores

It's as intense as the twenty-hour flight to Australia from nearly all points of North America. We love Blue Lizard because sun devotees have good reason to cover up with a very water-resistant sunscreen that lets you play hard and still stay sun-safe.

LOW Banana Boat Sunblock ($4)
Mass retailers

As a matter of fact, bananas are the number one selling item in grocery stores across America, and they may become scarce in the coming years. We can't save the bananas but we can save you from some serious skin damage by recommending Banana Boat products. They smell great and come in SPF 15, 30, and 50. For serious outdoor adventure, we also love the Banana Boat SPORT in SPF 30. It's ultrawaterproof and never feels greasy.

THE AUTHORS' PICK is the Banana Boat. You can find Banana Boat everywhere, it's inexpensive and it works. On top of this, it smells great!

After-sun Products

If there's one thing the Greeks know, it's how to have fun in the sun. Take a cue from them and don't forget to keep your after-sun products

---

BANANAS ARE GOOD FOR KIDS, TOO

Banana Boat Kids Tear Free SPF 30 is good for adults and kids. The antiburn system means you're virtually guaranteed the rays won't get through, and it's waterproof.

close at hand for when you might have gone just a little overboard. Korres after-sun products are designed to protect and repair skin damage from overexposure to the sun with the most natural ingredients for soothing effects.

HIGH Korres Yogurt Cooling Gel ($23)

www.searlenyc.com or www.korres.com

This cream-gel can be used on the face and body and has natural yogurt fat mixed in. The yogurt fat helps increase the water content at the top layers of the skin, instantly reviving UV-induced burning and redness. Fennel extract acts as an anti-inflammatory and anti-irritant, which helps promote healing in sun-harassed skin.

HIGH Korres Aloe Vera Moisturizing Body Milk ($23)

www.searlenyc.com or www.korres.com

Lightly textured and easily absorbed, this body lotion contains Active Aloe extract that soothes, heals, and relieves burned skin. Extracts of mimosa tenuiflora, a Mexican plant known for its ability to regenerate skin and promote cell renewal, and vitamin B$_5$ also deeply moisturize the skin and help relieve irritation.

HIGH Leaf & Rushner's Tx Night Cream ($75)

Bergdorf Goodman or call (888) 774-2424

This cream contains, and we love it when companies say this, "ground-breaking" DNA technology that acts like a morning-after pill for the skin. What this means is that it is actually able to reverse sun damage. It contains an enzyme that repairs DNA inside the skin cell that has been damaged by the sun and returns it to its original healthy state. This does not give you license to bake in the sun, but Tx Night Cream will greatly reduce the risk of long-term damage if you do!

Sun Hats
Physician Endorsed

By taking precautions, sun-worshipping fashionistas can enjoy the sun's warmth without the worry of wrinkles or sun damage. We love Physician Endorsed, a cutting-edge hat and accessories design company with fashionable and sun-safe accessories.

Physician Endorsed includes hats, sunglasses, and bags, all available with complimentary sunscreen and a photo tag showing how the hat should be worn. The hats are constructed with chemical-free fabrics and special linings to ensure the customer is receiving the highest-quality product, with a UPF rating of 50+ (equivalent to SPF 30). They're also handwashable and easy to pack! Prices range from $35 to $60, and they came in a variety of styles.

APPLY YOURSELF

Sun Mate Lotion Applicator solves the age-old dilemma, "How do I get the sunscreen on my back?" The hypolene pad won't absorb your lotion, oil, gel, or cream and keeps your hands clean so you can get those hard to reach places with ease. Available in four sun-fun colors ($6, www.Beautybuyble.com).

➤ For the sophisticate at the Sunday Polo match, the *Ginger*, a two-tone big brim style with reversible belt, is the ultimate accessory. Available in cotton candy/cactus, café/espresso, black/white, cornflower/vanilla, and white/black, the *Ginger* style provides the perfect protection.

➤ Flowers, flowers everywhere, for the girl with a green thumb. Keep yourself cool and protected while gardening with the *Barcelona* floral design. Featuring a large dramatic brim and round crown, this style is as essential as your gardening hose.

➤ The *St. Tropez*, featuring matching styles for "mommy and me," is ideal for a picnic with your little one. Help protect their delicate young skin and teach them sun protection early with this whimsical style available in cotton candy, cactus, pink lemonade, and aqua.

➤ For the poolside princess, the chic *Diva* style is the ideal accessory for lounging while sipping a daiquiri. This style offers a large brim to shield your face from the harsh effects of the sun, while keeping you looking simply fabulous.

SunStuff

SunStuff is another groovy company that makes sun hats. Founder Kathleen Burke was inspired to develop the headwear line several years ago, after her own search for a flattering sun protective hat to shield her Irish-American skin proved fruitless. She designed SunStuff hats to provide an effective and attractive solution to the mounting demand for serious sun protection. Although SunStuff carries products for men, women, and children, most of its products are designed by women for women, to ensure that the delicate balance between function and fashion is achieved. Its broad appeal has led to product requests from top-notch skin doctors at the Mayo Clinic and John Wayne Cancer Institute, fashion icons such as Vogue editor-in-chief Anna Wintour, and actresses such as Portia de Rossi, Allison Janney, and Amber Tamblyn. SunStuff products have appeared in *Cosmopolitan*, *Allure*, *Redbook*, *Self*, *Shape*, *Women's Health & Fitness*, *Better Homes and Gardens*, *Lucky*, and *Travel & Leisure* magazines. The company recently beat out 16,000 other applicants to win one of three grand prize winner spots in the 2004 Oxygen Network's "Build Your Business!" contest for hot women-owned companies.

Since not all hats are created equal, we posed a few questions to Kathleen Burke, founder of SunStuff Hats:

WHY IS A HAT SO NECESSARY DURING THE SUMMER MONTHS?

It is estimated that 90 percent of all aging of the skin—wrinkles, discoloration, and sagging—is attributable to sunlight, rather than to the passage of time. Americans are seeing cosmetic surgeons in droves to counteract the results of their sun-filled childhood days and the teen years baking in the sun with baby oil. Women spend billions of dollars each year on the creams they hope will repair and allay the visible damage to their skin. Skin cancer has reached epidemic proportions. The Mayo Clinic Medical Essay reports that almost half of all Americans who reach age sixty-five will develop skin cancer of one form or another, and reconstructive plastic surgery often follows removal of the offending cells.

Although publicity about the harmful effect of sun exposure has prompted many women to take better care of their skin, most women have a false sense of security arising from two myths: first, that sunscreen alone is effective at staving off skin damage, and second, that any hat will do the job. Although sunscreens are an essential part of sun protection, they are not effective alone. They rub and sweat off, they're hard to apply uniformly, and their protection doesn't last. You must wait at least twenty minutes before chemical sunscreens become effective by binding to the skin cells, and when sunblocks and sunscreens are active, the protection lasts only from twenty to eighty minutes. Finally, sunscreen blocks only some, not all, of the sun's damaging UV rays. Sunscreen is far more effective when coupled with a hat.

But not all hats are created equal in the battle against sun damage. Most hats are labeled "sun protective" as long as they have a 4-inch wide brim. A wide brim is not effective, however, if it is made of the straw or fabric found in most hats, which the sun's rays are able to penetrate. Hats made from typical lightweight fabrics, such as baseball hats and baby hats, allow up to 50 percent of harmful UVB rays (the equivalent of SPF 2 protection) and an even higher percentage of UVA rays through to the skin. If the fabric is damp or wet, as is often the case after workouts or near the water, it can transmit as much as 80 percent UVB radiation. Straw hats, depending on the weave, offer a similarly low level of protection.

WHAT MAKES SUNSTUFF HATS SO SPECIAL?

The company was launched in 2001 in response to the growing need of cosmetic surgeons and dermatologists for post-procedure protection that would effectively protect patients against sun-induced changes in the skin. Dermatologist Dr. Laurie Polis notes, "Women spend billions of dollars each year in an effort to reduce the wrinkling and spotting caused by sun damage. These changes to the skin are not inevitable. Sun protective clothing, like SunStuff UPF50+ products, used in conjunction with sunblock, helps prevent many signs of aging *before* they occur, so the skin is able to dedicate itself to the process of renewal rather than defense." SunStuff attempts to provide value as a permanent, day-to-day shield to protect youthful skin from wrinkles, spotting, and spider veins and appeal to those who are drawn to a fresh variety of styles. SunStuff hats not only met NASA's and the American Academy of Dermatology's standards for sun protection, but they are crushable, reversible, and hip.

I was inspired to develop a headwear line several years ago, after a search for a flattering sun-protective hat proved fruitless—the hats clearly were designed by men and targeted more for medical use, and lacked the pizzazz that women require from their accessories. The protective hats had no style, and the stylish hats offered no protection. Why shouldn't women have both sun protection and fashion in one hat?

SunStuff's state-of-the-art product line does what most hats do not—help preserve and protect youthful skin in three ways. First, the hats are designed for maximum facial and head coverage, with such features as downward-sloping, extended brims and protective, detachable face-shields, so that more skin is protected because less skin is exposed to direct sunlight. Second, they are made from UPF50+ sun protective fabric—designed to ensure that UVA ("aging") and UVB ("burning") rays are prevented from penetrating the hat and damaging the skin. And third, SunStuff knows that women will not consistently wear unattractive accessories no matter what the health benefit. Whether you want something traditional and elegant, or something trendy and fun, we've got you covered.

SHOULD CERTAIN STYLES BE WORN FOR CERTAIN OCCASIONS?

Hats should be worn any time women want to protect their skin from aging and damage. For day-to-day wear, a shorter brim is usually more acceptable, while for more formal occasions, a wider brim is appreciated. Of course, the width of brim is often dependent on the confidence level of the wearer.

Tanning Creams/ Lotions/ Bronzers

As we've discussed, the sun is not your best friend. On the other hand, you might not want to walk around with prison pallor either. You can still have a Cuban tan in your cubicle by using tanning creams, tanning lotions, and bronzers.

Tinted Body Moisturizers

The advantage to tinted moisturizers is that there's no risk involved. If you're even a tad bronze-shy, this is the way to go because the results are cumulative. So if you decide you don't like the slight difference, you simply stop moisturizing with these products.

HIGH DuWop Revolotion Tinted Body Moisturizer with SPF 15 and Shimmer ($21)
Mass retailers or Sephora stores

Call it crazy, call it weird, but whatever you call it, just don't ignore the hottest moisturizing trend: tinted body moisturizers that bring your pale up. This tinted moisturizer comes in three perfect shades for light, medium, and dark skin tones.

LOW Olay Body Touch of Sun Radiance Reviver ($7)
Drugstores

We love Olay so much that it's no wonder we love this product too. It's rich and moisturizing and provides the ever-so-slight darkening effect over time.

LOW Jergens Natural Glow Daily Moisturizer ($5.99)
www.walgreens.com

As the dark days of winter approach, a stress-free tanning situation is all you ask for. With the Jergens Natural Glow daily moisturizer you can finally stop tearing your hair out worrying about how you'll stay looking sunkissed through the cold, harsh winter. Jergens offers the perfect combination of subtle warming of your skin tone while staying perfectly moisturized.

THE AUTHORS' PICK is the Jergens. We love the way we don't have to argue with a self-tanner because of the streaks and lines, that there's no funky smell, and that our skin is perfectly moisturized as we slowly bake.

Body Tanners

HIGH Estée Lauder Self Tan Go Bronze Plus ($28.50)

www.esteelauder.com

This bronzer is dummy proof; it's tinted so you can see where you're putting it and it deepens over time. It also smells good, which is rare for bronzers.

HIGH Clarins Liquid Bronze Self Tanning ($29)

www.clarins.com

It goes on like milk and delivers an amazingly natural-looking tan every time. If you want to accessorize your itsy-bitsy bikini and look remarkably radiant for days, the Clarins is perfect for your holiday, any day.

MEDIUM Tantowel Self-Tan Towelettes Packets ($19.99)

Mass retailers

These little tan towels deliver impact that's overpowering, which is why we love them so much. You can travel with them so easily and whip one out whenever you need a professional polish or touch-up.

LOW Banana Boat Summer Color Sunless Instant Tanning Foam ($7)

Mass retailers

We love the lack of buttoned-up behavior of the Banana Boat brand. I mean seriously, the name is *Banana Boat,* and how fun is that? Furthermore, this sunless tanning foam is so easy to spread and nongreasy, which is also rare in the self-tanning category. It's also very lightweight and creates a beautiful golden nut of a tan. Also, the more often you apply, the deeper the tan.

LOW L'Oreal Sublime Bronze Self-Tanning Gelee ($9)

Mass retailers

It's not verboten to have a fake tan, but it is totally out of the question to have a tan that looks like a fake tan. L'Oreal is completely streak-free, dries quickly, and contains vitamin E and alpha hydroxy acids for smoother skin. More important, it leaves a gorgeous, rich, natural-looking tan, not that sweet potato look you may have worn in the 80s!

THE AUTHORS' PICK is the Banana Boat Tanning Foam because you can see it going on so you know exactly where you're putting it to avoid streaks and it sets up nicely. It's also cheap.

Tanners for the Face

"Not in the face!" Yeah, that's what your last wussy boyfriend screamed just as you discovered all those suspicious calls on his cell phone. Unwittingly, the lout was giving you

RX FOR COOL CHICKS

L'Oreal Solar Expertise Milk Spray-Mist is a great coolant if you start to sizzle in the sun. It contains fine particles of milk, which soothe burning skin, and an SPF of 15. ($19, only available through www .auravita.com).

good advice—you do need to be careful with your face. You may want to get that tan sun-kissed look without wasting the time in passé tanning salons or spending the money on that real weekend in the Bahamas. But you need to exercise caution and use self-tanners specifically designed for the face, or you risk the "muddy look"—looking like the victim of a particularly sloppy "swirly." Worse, you could end up with a really uncool orange face, and that's so Oompa-loompa 1971.

HIGH Clarins Tinted Self Tanning Face Cream SPF 15 ($28)

Department stores or www.sephora.com

The most exertion you'll feel getting this tan is applying it to the face. In just two hours a natural, sun-kissed glow appears. It also has an SPF 15 to keep you covered anytime you're outdoors.

HIGH Dior Bronze Self-Tanner for Face ($26)

Department stores or www.sephora.com

If you love a little bronze over a little brown, this is the perfect replica of a natural bronze. It sets up in just a few hours and lasts through the dance-off.

MEDIUM Origins Faux Glow radiant self-tanner for face ($17.50)

Department stores or www.origins.com

There's no sun in sight, but who's to know with the right self-tanner? Sun-craved skin looks and feels pretty and remarkably radiant for days with Origins. And the tinted formula delivers an instant coulda-fooled-me tan that shows what you've done and still need to do (this way you never streak or stripe). The added perk: the refreshing aroma of peppermint.

THE AUTHORS' PICK is the Clarins, because it smells great, moisturizes, and contains SPF 15 for good sun protection.

HEAD-TO-TOE SELF-TANNING TIPS

Rita Ukis, esthetician at Avon Salon & Spa adores a well applied tan. As one of the *Beauty Buyble* experts, we asked Rita to enlighten us on how to apply an A-list look that is, (whisper it) anything but barely there.

1. Exfoliate prior to applying self-tanner to the body. This allows the color to be absorbed more evenly.
2. Make sure your body is completely dry or the cream will not absorb. You should also be completely naked to assure complete and even coverage.
3. Apply self-tanner using a very thin, surgical latex glove to prevent the color from staining your hands and fingers.
4. Starting with your feet and legs, glide quarter-size amounts of self-tanner in an upward sweeping motion, avoiding the knuckles and joints where the tanners typically set in darker. After you finish with one

TAN PRESERVATION

Shaving cannot remove a natural tan, but it will slough away dead skin that is pigmented with a fake tan. Reapply your tanning creams, lotions, or sprays after shaving to freshen up the color.

area, use only what is left on the gloves to go over knuckles and joints.

5. Moving up to the hips and waist area, continue with a palm full of tanner, blending up around your belly and chest area in a circular motion. It is best to have someone else do your back to ensure a smooth transition of color.

6. Continue sweeping upward on your neck. For the face, put a dime-sized amount of self-tanner on gloves to go over the face, being careful to thin out sparingly around the eyes, lips and ears. If you wear your hair up in the summer, be sure to get behind the ear and sweep toward the hairline.

7. If you mess up, use a Q-tip dipped in alcohol or nail polish remover to sweep over toenails and in the nail grooves to soak up color clumps.

8. Your faux tan will not protect you from the sun, and the exfoliation will make your skin more photosensitive! Apply sunscreen liberally once your self-tanner has set (about four hours), and at least a half hour before going into the sun.

Spray Tanning Formulations

The best sprays come in quick-dry aerosol formulas to deliver a superfine mist that doesn't force you to have to rub it in; helping you to avoid streaking. For best results, spray while moving the can rapidly across your skin. If you stay in one place too long you can have a heavier demarcation in that region, a dead giveaway that you weren't actually in St. Tropez.

HIGH MODEL℠ Tan Airbrush in a Can ($36)
Select Victoria's Secret or Sephora stores

If you want to escape the tedium of wondering how dark you'll actually get with a spray-on tan, the MODEL℠ Tan Airbrush in a Can is for you. The deep, golden color is immediate and if you hold the spray in any one place for a longer period of time the color is markedly darker. We only caution that you do need to keep a solid sweeping motion because it goes on so dark that if you concentrate in any one area for too long you'll have spots. It also has a yummy cocoa butter scent!

MEDIUM Clarins Self Tanning Instant Spray ($29)
Fine department stores or www.sephora.com

Beachbreak: Lots of jetties and a curving coast mean you have to rip to be part of the beautiful people. Just don't forget your Clarins Self Tanning Instant Spray before you suit up to surf. It will allow you to hit the surf scene with a lovely bronze

MARATHON MOISTURE

Put your moisturizer on steroids with DHC Mild Lotion ($28, www.dhccare.com). It's a revitalizing tonic that helps your moisturizer go the extra mile to keep your skin fresh and hydrated. It's also alcohol-free and contains cucumber juice that soothes the skin.

and moisturizes your skin just in time for those saltwater waves.

LOW **Neutrogena MicroMist Tanning Sunless Spray ($12)**
Mass retailers

If the goal is to glean a light, natural-looking tan in a flash, you'll love the Neutrogena. The proletarian price tag is a draw, but this is an alcohol-free aerosol, so it won't dry the skin, and goes on oh so evenly.

THE AUTHORS' PICK is the MODEL^{co} Tan Airbrush in a Can, because you can achieve a very quick bronzed glow that intensifies in hours and fades naturally without streaking.

Bar Soap

An often overlooked part of any beauty regimen is soap—yes, good old-fashioned soap. What is the point of all the creams, lotions, and makeup if you're just going to use a sub-par generic soap on skin that you've worked so hard to make soft and beautiful? Using the right soap will help you maintain beautiful and healthy skin, and ladies, it takes great raw materials to make great art.

LOW **Vitabath Gelee Bar Soap ($5)**
Department stores

The Vitabath soaps are packed with lots of do-good properties like vitamins A, D, and E; sunflower oil; and horse chestnut extract. You can't resist the Original Spring Green scent, but it does come in three other invigorating palettes: Plus for Dry Skin, Fresh Citrus Twist, and Spa Skin Therapy.

LOW **Palmer's Cocoa Butter Formula Cream Soap ($2)**
Mass retailers

Palmer's is the doyenne of dollar stores, and yet this old-timer reigns supreme in so many categories. Soaps are tricky because some of us have allergies and can't use just any soap. But you won't have that problem with Palmer's; it's vitamin E rich, gentle, and won't leave you with that tight feeling that so many soaps do.

LOW **Dove Beauty Bars ($7 for a package of six)**
Mass retailers

To avoid the peculiar mélange of body odors next time you hop on the subway or find yourself trapped in an elevator six deep, Dove steps in to keep you fresh as a daisy, so that the only vintage you notice is your own special blend.

BLACK DIAMOND TRUFFLES ANYONE?

This is an ultraluxurious body butter that is made with real imported black diamond truffles, which are the most expensive and sought after truffles in France and Italy. Black Diamond Truffle is available from Selona Beauty (www.selonabeauty.com) in a body butter, exfoliating body scrub, and pure moisture body wash. $50 for 4 ounces.

LOW Blooming Grove Soap ($4.50)

www.bloominggrove.net

In a rare display of invention, Jennifer Urezzio has created soaps and other customized beauty products to combine cleanliness of the body and mind. Her products are fused with organically grown herbs and oils, intended to nurture the body and delight the soul. So whether you're just plain getting clean or you need a little personality adjustment, you're sure to find a Blooming Grove soap that will do the job.

THE AUTHORS' PICK is the Vitabath. Often overlooked in the drugstore, it seems like it's been around for centuries—our mothers and even our grandmothers used it. We love it because it keeps on giving the same fresh, clean feeling we expect.

Body Creams/ Lotions

If you want to stop the raging of the aging you need the motion of the lotion. Oils and lotions hydrate your skin and keep it looking and feeling young and soft. Every woman should work some lotion time into her schedule—and if it comes with a massage, all the better! We are positively ga ga about body creams and lotions, so we've listed as many as we could here.

OUTRAGEOUS Trish McEvoy Super Enriched Body Cream ($48)

www.neimanmarcus.com

Unfortunately for your pocketbook, this is just the most divine body cream ever. It smells like blackberry, and goes on so richly and smoothly that you'll find yourself compulsively applying it without even noticing time passing by.

OUTRAGEOUS Inara Babassu Body Crème ($44)

www.inaraorganic.com

A good strategy against dry skin can secure victory. Babassu Body Crème will demonstrate all the reasons you need the right moisturizer because it works so well. It's also 100 percent organic and has an olive oil base for exceptional penetrating power.

HIGH Bliss Naked Body Butter ($32)

Bliss Spa locations, www.blissworld.com, or (888) 243-8825

Ever wonder just how far beauty companies will go to satisfy a demanding woman? Bliss has taken out the fragrance from their bestselling tube of skin tenderizing moisturizer for those who don't wish to surrender to perfumey products. Fragrance-phobes, drop your robes!

MEDIUM CeraVe Moisturizing Cream ($14.99)

Mass retailers

MAD ABOUT MUD

Borghese Fango Active Mud ($32, 7 ounces) for face and body is a superb all-over body mask. It detoxifies the skin and improves skin tone, and we swear it takes a few inches off the thighs if you use it regularly (www.nordstrom.com).

While you don't want 30 percent more added to your tush, a thicker, more formidable moisturizing cream is good for chapped, cracked, and dry skin, and this one packs a punch. The CeraVe lotion is lighter weight and fragrance-free ($12.99).

LOW NIVEA Soft ($2.99)
Mass retailers

NIVEA Soft is so, so, soft—like a baby's bottom or the tummy of a kitten. It's a light-textured cream that has a whipped, soufflé-like texture and gives the skin a uniquely, well, soft feeling. It's not greasy, it absorbs quickly, it's ultrahydrating and it's, did we say, soft? Try it and you'll be addicted!

LOW NIVEA Crème ($1 to $7)
Mass retailers

NIVEA Crème is both soft and creamy, like a Krispy Kreme crème-filled donut, only rubbing NIVEA on won't make you fat. Oh, and we're not inflating the results.

THE AUTHORS' PICK for Maureen is the Trish McEvoy, because the smell is heavenly and it's just such a decadent moisturizer. The Authors' Pick for Paula is the NIVEA Soft. At this price you can buy as much as you like, as often as you like, guilt free.

In Shower Body Wash

It's now the twenty-first century. We don't use pay phones. We don't pop in a VHS tape. We get nostalgic over old movies of a gentler time like *Jerry Maguire* and *There's Something about Mary*. We take strolls down memory lane by doing such anachronistic pastimes as washing with soap. But times have moved on. The civilized world has developed body washes to make sure every bit and bob gets clean. These multihued liquids are lighter and produce far more fluffy lather without a filmy residue (that's just *so* twentieth century), and many are scented with fragrances that you'd be proud to wear out in public.

HIGH Philosophy Amazing Grace Foaming Bath and Shower Gel ($22)
Department stores

The scent is so pure and fresh you will leave the shower craving your next wash. For the price there is also a generous amount of product, which is one reason we love the Philosophy body washes.

JELLYBATH

The most exciting new bath soak, foot soak, and hand soak is Jellybath (www.jellybath.com). It's a patented technology that literally changes the viscosity of water and retains heat four times longer than regular water. It reduces swelling, lowers blood pressure, relaxes muscles, and exfoliates and softens the skin just like a sauna. Just add Jellybath to warm water and it becomes a translucent, fluffy jelly—a virtual bath blanket—that cradles you in luxury. To get the goo down the drain, add the second packet of salt and it dissolves the Jellybath instantly. Now how's that for invention?

LOW **Skin So Soft Light & Lush Creamy Body Wash ($6.99)**

www.avon.com

Paula,

My knickers are positively in a bunch over Avon's Skin So Soft Light & Lush Creamy Body Wash. After a five-mile hike through the mountains of Utah I couldn't break free fast enough for a hot shower. I'd forgotten my soap—you know how I forget to pack ANYthing when I travel—but one of the other writers on the trip had an extra bottle of the Avon body wash. Now that I've tried it I know why she always carries two bottles—you can't put it down and oh, what a night of blissful zzzs.

—Maureen

PS: The SSS Light & Lush Shower Gel is designed with a hook so it hangs from your shower—woo hoo!

LOW **Palmer's Cocoa Butter Formula Moisturizing Body Wash ($3.19)**

Mass retailers

While not exactly a shower gel or a lotion, we cannot ignore the generosity of this product; the creamy, nonsoap formula produces a seemingly never-ending rich lather that moisturizes while cleansing.

Shower Gels

Shower gels? Well, we were going to direct you back to the chapter on Body Washes, but our editor reminded us that we have a contract for so many words for this book, and that the publisher won't pay us unless we reach and slightly exceed that number. So we're going to vamp here for a few minutes—just as if we were on a

A WORD FROM FIJI

Pure Fiji has created a menu of products based on authentic South Pacific island rituals. Cold-pressed virgin coconut oil, coconut milk, and exotic nut extracts form the basis for the Pure Fiji spa products line, produced in Suva, Fiji. Similar to the high-quality virgin olive oil found in a gourmand's kitchen, virgin coconut oil is hand-pressed cold from fresh coconuts in order to retain the most natural nutrients. Products in the collection contain herbs found in the Fiji islands. Here are just a few of our favorites:

➤ Pure Fiji Coconut Milk Bath Soak

➤ Pure Fiji Passionflower Body Butter

➤ Pure Fiji Starfruit Hydrating Lotion

➤ Pure Fiji Mana'ia Body Butter

Celebrities such as Denise Richards, Nicole Kidman, Rachel Hunter, and Taye Diggs are all fans of Pure Fiji's line of natural products, which are available online at www.purefiji.com as well as at select retailers nationwide such as Barney's New York, Palmetto, and the Studio at Fred Segal.

bad date, killing time until dessert and. . . . Hmm. It's not working. In truth, there is a small difference between shower gels and body washes, it lies in the consistency or feel of the product. Shower gels typically have a thinner consistency and can be drying. Also, the creamier body washes tend to lather up faster. It's two slightly different roads that essentially get you to the same place: clean.

HIGH Naturopathica Zesty Lime Shower Gel ($32)

Leading spas and resorts, (800) 669-7618 or www.naturopathica.com

You might get confused with this shower gel, which harkens the scents of Mia Moana island in French Polynesia, but don't worry, it's just Naturo-pathica doing what it does best; takes you far, far away with enticing aromas. This invigorating gel contains extracts of nettle, meadowsweet, and milk thistle to hydrate the skin and aloe vera and sweet almond protein to maintain the skin's lipid barrier. The blend of lime, blood orange, and ginger is fresh and enlivening. It would probably also make a great smoothie.

MEDIUM Vitabath Spa Skin Therapy Bath & Shower Gelee ($28)

Drugstores

Vitabath offers the bath and shower gelee in several varieties, including Original Spring Green,

Plus for Dry Skin, Fresh Citrus Twist, and the Spa Skin Therapy. Whatever your preferences, you'll be delighted to reunite with this old favorite.

LOW Avon Skin So Soft Shower Gel ($2.99)

(800) for-Avon or www.avon.com

Your grandmother probably still has a bottle of Avon Skin So Soft oil sitting around somewhere, and damn that's an old bottle of SSS. She loved it when she was younger for good reason, and to-day we've graduated to an expanded line of SSS products that include the shower gel, which delivers the same signature softening benefits with a fantastic aroma.

THE AUTHORS' PICK is the Vitabath, because it smells so great, it has the right price tag, and the brand is an old reliable.

Body Exfoliators

There's no pretty way to put this. Body exfolia-tors remove all the dead skin and dirt from your epidermis. Ew. It's like a snake that sheds its old skin, for a brand new shiny one. Double ew. But that's what these do, and they are important in your beauty routine to keep

MUST-HAVE MOISTURE

Olay Moisturinse In Shower Body Lotion revolutionizes body moisturization, working in the shower to condition skin in the privacy of your own shower. At $4.99 or $6.99 for a larger bottle, this is a *Beauty Buyble* "aha!" moment you can't miss.

MORE THAN MOISTURIZERS

All-natural products that fulfill multiple moisturizing needs are a big trend this year. Indigo **Zum Rub** is the perfect skinny-dipping edition to your moisturizing wardrobe. Zum Rub cures hangnails, dry heels, cuts, chapped lips, frizzy hair, and much much more. Zum is an all-natural, nonmineral oil moisturizer with goat's milk, shea butter, essential oils, and aromatherapy. Even better, it soaks in easily but doesn't clog pores. It comes in almond, frankincense & myrrh, lavender, patchouli, rosemary, mint, and tea tree citrus ($9, www.indigowild.com).

your skin soft and fresh, with the additional use of oils and lotions. The good news is, unless you are dating Hannibal Lecter, your chances of becoming a really cool belt or pair of shoes in the future is much less than the snake's.

OUTRAGEOUS Inara Enliven Sugar Rub ($65)
www.inaraorganic.com

Forget Pilates. Recharge with this luxurious rub. By massaging the Sugar Rub onto wet skin then rinsing thoroughly, preferably in a rain forest, the skin emerges feeling more vibrant and soft than ever. The rare combination of native turbinado sugar and babassu oil gently exfoliates and conditions, and for the price tag you get a beautiful custom crock for mixing.

HIGH Selona Exfoliating Body Scrub ($45)
www.selonabeauty.com

Pure sugar, rich oils, and sexy skin . . . oh my! Your fella will flip over the irresistible way your skin feels, and your bonus is getting rid of the dead skin on your body without that greasy after-feeling many scrubs have. Our favorite is the Black Diamond Truffle body scrub because, first you gotta love a company that imports black diamond truffles from France and Italy just to sell it to you in a scrub that you wash down your drain, and let's face it, where else will you ever find anything close to a diamond next to your skin?

MEDIUM Vitabath Exfoliating Sugar Scrub ($17.50)
Drugstores

Even if you climb out of bed on Sunday morning and throw on your boyfriend's jeans you'll feel sexy as hell after a bout with Vitabath Sugar Scrub. While there are four exciting scents for the sugar scrub, the Plus for Dry Skin is a fave be-

SOFT SPOT

Palmer's Cocoa Butter Formula Swivel Stick ($3, mass retailers) is an awesome on-the-spot moisturizer for anything: chapped lips, blemishes, or any area of the body that seems rough, cracked, or dry. We love to butter up with this product.

cause it soothes dry skin with a mysterious, romantic scent while you exfoliate, and it never stings when used after shaving.

THE AUTHORS' PICK is the Inara Sugar Rub. It's expensive, we know, but the packaging and product can't be beat and let's face it, there's something very Willy Wonka about rubbing sugar all over your body from a chocolate-colored pot.

Hand Creams/Lotions

Eyes may be the windows to the soul, but hands are a window into your age. Close that window. Your hands are always working and almost an afterthought on a busy day, but hand care is important. There's little point in having the face of an angel and a body of a teenager if your crone-like claws are going to give you away. Use hand creams and lotions frequently, and if you remember to use ones with SPF, all the better. Work that pump several times a day so your hands stay creamy and dreamy for years into the future. That way, your hands will never tell tales on you.

HIGH Rich Girl Therapeutic Hand and Cuticle Cream ($24)

Sephora, Bergdorf Goodman, Neiman Marcus, or Nordstrom

Totally rich babes don't have dark spots or pigmentation on their hands. Why? Hellooooo, they know the rich girl secret: NEVER EVER LEAVE HOME WITHOUT SUNSCREEN ON YOUR HANDS! The UVA/UVB SPF 25 sun protection in this product will make it seem like you're a rich girl even if you're not.

MEDIUM Yu-Be Moisturizing Skin Cream ($15)

www.yu-be.com

If the creamsicle colors and Japanese characters on the tube aren't enough to reel you in, then perhaps the fact that this is the must-have cream for world-class mountain climbers on Mt. Everest will. It keeps their roughest spots buttery soft without the residual grease from most hand creams and lotions. We also hear that it's done wonders for people with eczema and dermatitis.

BATH FROM THE PAST

We remember the old slogan, "Calgon, Take Me Away," but who knew they were still around? Oh yes, and better than ever. Don't pinch yourself—you're not dreaming. You can spritz any time you like and for extra cool sensations, keep it in the fridge, and feel the Caribbean Sea wash over your senses. For additional tropical paradise, try the Calgon Tropical Dream Moisture Rich Shower & Bath Gel ($5.25). It's luxurious and soap-free, yet gently cleanses and is loaded with skin conditioners that are quickly absorbed. The Tropical Dream Body Lotion ($5.25) glides on smoothly to soothe even the most sensitive skin and the Tropical Dream Body Mist ($6.95) will leave you feeling fresh and revitalized, just as you might upon the return from your dream vacation. Available at mass retailers.

LOTION-PHOBES REJOICE!

We also love the Vitabath Moisturizing Dry Oil Spray ($12.95, drugstore.com). If you're a tad lotion-phobic, or you just don't like excess lotion on your skin, say maybe in the summer when it's hot, the dry oil spray is the perfect elixir.

LOW Eucerin Original Moisturizing Lotion and Creme ($4.99–$11.99)

Mass retailers

Eucerin is ideal for the girl who wants a no-nonsense approach to moisturization. Whether you're a cream lover or a lotion-o-file, you will never be disappointed with Eucerin. It's fragrance free, won't clog pores, and works on all skin types.

THE AUTHORS' PICK is even-handed. We both love the Yu-Be and have been wondering where it's been all our lives.

Perfect Nails

There's nothing better than treating yourself to a professional manicure or pedicure. But you can save money by doing it yourself at home. These tips will take your nails from ragged to refined in no time.

Start with Ms. Manicure

A salon manicure takes time and money. If neither works for you, take this insider tip and invest instead in Ms. Manicure's top-notch nail care tools to transform nails from apprentices to divas. Here are our favorites:

➤ A portable nail salon, **Ms. Manicure At-Your-Fingertips** kit ($12.99) has all the essentials in a compact vinyl case with two zippered pockets, one for tools and the other for your fave polishes.
➤ Go mini with the **Marvelous Mini** Smoothing and Shaping kit ($2.99), which contains tiny tools that deliver full-size power.
➤ **Ms. Manicure Folding 4-way Nail Buffer** ($1.49) gives four ways to make nails sensational; one side shapes the nail, another smooths. Flip to buff and polish nails to velvety matte finish.

GERM-A-PHOBES REJOICE!

Jao hand refresher is a sanitizer with essential oils, which eliminates that dry feeling you get with most sanitizers. Instead, you get the wonderful scent of lavender and chamomile combined with sage, geranium, and eucalyptus. It's like a cup of cream tea for your hand ($7, www.productjunkies.com).

➤ Night out and the nail goes wild? Whip out a **Ms. Manicure Quick Fix**: twelve emery boards in a matchbook to slip in pockets and tiny purses (.99).

➤ Why are emery boards hard, stiff, sandy, and brown? **Ms. Manicure Washable Emery Boards** ($1.99) are cushy and flexible, to bend easily to shape oval or square nails. They do double-duty with a medium texture on one side to shape. Flip to the fine texture for an extra-smooth finish.

➤ Don't hang around with hangnails. Clip, snip, but never tear or pull precious nails with the **Ms. Manicure Nail Clipper** ($1.49). The nonslip, rubber grip and ergonomic shape lets you size up too long or mismatched nails, hand to toe.

➤ ER for nails: **Ms. Manicure Just in Case** kit ($10.99) is for fast first-aid. It includes nail glue, acetone corrector pen, shine-n-go, buffer, and more.

Cuticle Creams

Beauty Buyble girls may, in their spare time, drive eighteen wheelers, smoke big old stogies, play mud football, and even throw darts, but they do it while looking like they're ready for a red carpet walk, at any moment. The trick? Attention to details. One small detail that removes a lot of "ick" is cuticle care. A quality cuticle cream softens your cuticles and makes them easy to keep trim and tidy, not thick, dry, and flaky. That way, your friends will believe that you just came back from a stint on the runways of Paris or Milan, and not your taxidermy club weekend in Petersville, Montana.

HIGH **Nailtiques Cuticle and Hand Conditioner ($12.99)**
drugstore.com

This fabulous cream transforms simple hands to works of art. It contains a highly concentrated combination of pure aloe and jojoba oils that rehydrates and conditions the hands and cuticle area.

LOW **Sally Hansen Diamond Strength Cuticle and Nail ($5.95)**
Drugstores

Perseverance works! We searched high and low to find a great nail oil and cuticle cream in one, and here we have it. This cuticle and nail oil is instantly absorbed into the nail—unlike many that sit on the surface and feel greasy—and bathes the nail with grape seed oil, lavender, and protein. Use regularly and you'll reveal a healthier, stronger nail.

LOW **Burt's Bees Lemon Butter Cuticle Cream ($3.25–$4.99)**
Specialty outlets or www.burtsbees.com

This cream is not only affordable, it appeals to traditionalists and bohemians alike who write to the company in praise of the small wonder. The lemon oil softens your cuticles and strengthens your nails at the same time. The company boasts that you can even use it on your toe cuticles!

THE AUTHORS' PICK is the Burt's Bees. We love the way it smells and softens, and gives a luxury skin-care treatment at a pauper's price.

Base Polish

Without a decent base polish for your nails you are on the fast-track to fashionably dead. Without a good base polish, your nail polish will slip right off and sing "sayonara" on its way down your slacks. The secret to success lies in the base.

HIGH   Embellish Transforming Seal for Nails ($8.50)

Fine salons

The sparkly sealant blends with nail color to totally obscure chips and imperfections. It also transforms rough, rigid nails into smooth slopes.

MEDIUM   Seche Base ($7)

www.prosalonsupply.com

Forget crystal balls and wise up to the fact that to land a man you're going to need great hair, great skin, a super-duper wardrobe, and nails that say "the world is my oyster." Seche Vite's technology delivers stronger, healthier nails that will have him turning over those property deeds and stock portfolios well before you hit Portofino.

LOW   Sally Hansen Diamond Strength Base & Top Coat ($5.95)

Drugstores

Sally Hansen always tops the highest bar for innovation. The diamond's strength is combined here with optimal shine in a very quick-drying product that doesn't chip. It gives up to ten days of wear as a base or top coat.

LOW   NUTRINE Garlic Nail Hardener ($3.79)

harmondiscount.com

All artists know that you have to prime your medium before applying paint. This garlic base coat naturally fortifies your nails to make the nail stronger and healthier, allowing the top coat to really shine and draw attention to your beautiful fingernails, rather than just attempt to cover up your claws. And Bonus! With pungent garlic extract in the nail polish itself, it will severely curtail your desire to ever pick your nose.

THE AUTHORS' PICK is the Sally Hansen. We just cannot ignore the fact that nothing penetrates Sally. Nothing, ever. And at $5.95 that's some serious security.

EXPERT TIPS FOR KNOCKOUT NAILS

Steven Vu, owner of the Dallas-based L.A. Nail & Spa, shared two important salon secrets with *The Beauty Buyble:*

➤ When you're getting your nails done in a nail salon, be sure to ask if they use the most effective sanitation process for their nail tools. This includes both soaking the tools in a disinfectant and placing them in a sterilization pouch for each and every nail service.

NAIL TREATMENTS WE LOVE

➤ FACE Stockholm Nail Food. FACE Stockholm has some of the primo products on the beauty market and this cuticle food is fabulous. It contains sesame oil, lavender, and myrrh.

➤ Creative Nail Design Systems SolarOil. This product has jojoba oil, vitamin E, and almond oil. Check it out.

➤ Decleor Nail Treatment Oil. This cuticle softener has essential oils of myrrh, lemon, and parsley.

SAVE THOSE NAILS!

Moisturize and repair the toughest nails with the Nail Saver ($6.99, www.amazon.com). The unique formula brightens nails, saving them from discoloration, and gives them a crystal clear appearance.

➤ **A salon technician should always apply two layers of nail polish. The color will not be rich enough with one coat; more than two coats will make the polish chip easily. Balance is the key.**

Nail Polish

Did you know that the only word in the English language that changes its pronounation with a capital letter is polish? Yes, we at the *Beauty Buyble* spend many hours working hard to bring you important facts like that. Next year we might even do a section on Nail Polish (we hear Warsaw is lovely in the spring), but this year we have a very limited budget for travel, so we'll just have to make do with this section on nail polish.

Nail polish (small "p") is important. Yes, it protects the nails, yada, yada, yada. More importantly, it completes the beauty circle—

a girl's nails say a great deal about her. It tells you if she's tasteful and sophisticated, if she's vibrant and fun, or it will tattle on her if she's a complete mess. Selecting good nail polish is key in any good beauty circle.

HIGH **Chanel Le Vernis Nail Colour ($18)**
Fine department stores

The Chanel nail colors are absolutely the deepest, richest, and most beautiful polish shades ever developed. They are so signature that you can truly recognize a Chanel shade when it's on someone else. The bottles are ingeniously designed so that they don't spill, and the lacquer hugs your nails with strengtheners and moisturizers.

MEDIUM **lippmann *collection* ($15)**
www.lippmanncollection.com

With names like Just Walk Away Renee, a berry black cherry for Renee Zellweger; Sarah Smile, a sheer, sexy pink for Sarah Jessica Parker; What-

PROPER PREPARATION

Celebrity manicurist Karla Cay advises the following for nail prepping: first file and shape the nails, remove cuticles with a cuticle remover, push back gently on the nail bed, then apply a cuticle oil to rehydrate the cuticles. Use a soft two-sided buffer to smooth out the nail bed, then take a nail brush with soap and water to remove oils from nail bed. This will allow the polish to stay much longer. MAKE SURE YOU USE A BASECOAT. It helps protect the nail bed from staining that icky yellow and allows virtually any brand of nail polish to stay put.

QUICK STRIP

e.l.f. Nail Polish Remover Pads are killer! We've tried so many handy on-the-go nail polish remover pads and we can't believe our good fortune with e.l.f. Like every other e.l.f. product, they are only $1, and they strip your nails faster than a Brazillian wax at rush hour.

ever Lola Wants, a sparkly, pale pink for Kelly Ripa's daughter Lola, there's a lot of diva charm behind Lippmann's trend-setting colors. The polish is quick-drying and contains all kinds of extra-fun ingredients, such as green tea extracts, which help build biotin for strong nails.

MEDIUM MAC Nail Lacquer ($9)

www.maccosmetics.com

MAC Nail Lacquer boasts a revolutionary new high-gloss formula; it's a no-streak and no-chip finish. Three finishes—cream, sheer, and frosted—give you a candy store of options within the color spectrum, and each contains UV protection so that the color won't sour when you're at the beach!

LOW Sally Hansen Diamond Strength No Chip Nail Color ($4.79)

Mass retailers

Day Seven: After lunch onboard the Ivana *I settle into my usual sunbathing routine and notice*

my nails. I'm wearing Sally Hansen Diamond Strength nail color, Lavender Marquis, and it looks the same as the day I left for the Grand Cayman Islands. How can this be? I've been plunging into the deep azure waters, swimming in private pools at various ports of call, sunbathing for hours, exposing my hands to the UV rays, and working product after product through my sun-soaked hair. All this and no chipping, no fading? Diamond strength, diamond shine, diamond wear. They're not kidding.

—Paula's travel diary

e.l.f. Color Protection Nail Lacquer ($1)

www.elfcosmetics.com

The cold air snapped as we scurried through the snow from our Hum-V to the cabin in Woodstock, Vermont. My husband, Will, was surprising me with an extended weekend getaway, and I was prepared—even though I had no idea where

GOODNESS GRACIOUS, IT'S GOLDIE!

While not necessarily the longest lasting, we can't resist Goldie Nail Lacquers because they are packaged in these darling petite yet curvy bottles, blossoming under a delicate flower cap with a white ribbon tied around the bottle. So girlie, so feminine. We also love the shades: Cashy, Creepy, Groovy, Bunny, 80s, Charlie, Rumors, Tackquoi, Cheap, Gelee, Pillow, Lost, Veil, Rapture, Pansy, Wulung, and Paradis. $9, Bath & Body Works flagship stores nationwide.

we were going exactly. Before we headed off for the six-hour drive, I glossed my fingernails with e.l.f. nail lacquer in Marie's Hot Rod, a deep wine that just so happened to go with the Bordeaux and box of Debauve & Gallais chocolates waiting for us by the fireplace. Skiing, snow-shoeing, and maple sugaring were no challenge to this polish.

—*Maureen's travel diary*

THE AUTHORS' PICK is the Sally Hansen Diamond Strength. This is serious industrial-strength nail polish. It lasts for two weeks plus and never chips, and the color selections are amazing.

Top Coat

Wear, watch, read, listen, and look. You don't go out of the house with dark roots, right? And we know you don't go to bed at night with makeup on, right? The eleventh commandment—the one that was edited out in earlier buyble study groups—is, "You shall not wear nail polish without a top coat." Why? Because we said so. No, really, because the top coat seals in the layers beneath it. It makes sure your nail polish stays put and shines like the moon on steroids. A top coat is an essential *Beauty Buyble* girl must.

Seche Vite Fast Dry Top Coat ($10)

www.prosalonsupply.com

Top coats are basically colorless nail polish with a higher degree of solvent to evaporate more quickly. Seche Vite creates a reaction like an epoxy resin—it penetrates the nail polish and fuses all the layers, compacting them into one coating, thus no chipping and peeling. It also contains UV protectants and creates a single solid, clear shield that the sun cannot penetrate.

MEDIUM Lippmann Collection "On a Clear Day" Top Coat ($16)

www.lippmancollection.com

You just have to have a UV light inhibitor for a top coat that won't turn gray, and this one has it. It also dries very quickly and is ultra glossy.

LOW Poshe TopCoat ($9.49)

www.poshe.com

Poshe Top Coat contains no toluene, an ingredient that makes most top coats simply cover and dry when applied over nail polish. When Poshe Top Coat is applied over your existing manicure, it blends with and rewets the old polish. This will remove any surface scratches and dissolve the oxidation, returning the color to its original shade. It will revive the gloss with Poshe's award-winning shine, the highest available.

LOW Sally Hansen Diamond Strength Base & Top Coat ($5.95)

Mass retailers

NO SHY NAILS

Bright colors reign for summer. Madonna, Julianne Moore and Alicia Silverstone love Chanel Le Vernis nail colour collection. Hot pink and hot coral are reminiscent of exotic, sandy, sun-drenched seascapes.

LOW **Out the Door Top Coat ($3.99)**

Beauty suppliers

Celebrity manicurist Karla Cay turned us on to this amazing top coat. The name says it all—one application and you have a super-shiny coat that is dry nearly as fast as your brush leaves the nail. Karla suggests adding an extra top coat to nails two days after your manicure to bring back the shine and keep the polish on.

THE AUTHORS' PICK is the Sally Hansen because if you haven't learned by now, *we love sally.*

NAILS WITH STAYING POWER

Celebrity manicurist Karla Cay gives us some super tips to helping your manicure last.

➤ **Wash and dry hands first. Prepare nail surface using polish remover to remove any oil or lotion.**

➤ **Apply a Toluene-free base coat such as Seche Vite ($7, www.prosalonsupply.com) to a thoroughly dry nail.**

➤ **Apply two coats of polish, sweeping lightly and quickly from the base to the edge.**

➤ **Let the polish dry thoroughly between coats.**

FABULOUS FINGERS AND TANTALIZING TOES

Skyy Hadley of As U Wish Nail Spa in Hoboken, New Jersey, gives the following tips to keep your fingers and toes in fashion:

➤ *Shimmers are back big time*. Light shades look best in summer, so make sure they have a shimmer to them. Shimmer polishes add sexiness to nails that matte shades miss.

➤ *Round nails are the shape*. The square shape is over. But if you're too afraid of the full-fledged round nail, go for the squoval (a little round, a little square) look to test the waters.

➤ *Add a little dazzle*. We're starting to see jewels again, especially on toes. But it has to be done right—a cute little flower on one foot centered with a gem is classy; a whole toe of dazzle is just crazy. Think dainty, not diva.

➤ *In-salon versus at-home*. See your manicurist every two months, especially for toes, but in-between touch-ups at home are easy and convenient. Be sure to change polish when it is chipped, and if you are filing nails, try to follow the shape that your manicurist has already given you. In addition, keep hands and feet well moisturized and they'll look young and healthy.

➤ ***Keep feet fresh.*** Fill a spritzer bottle with a mixture of lemon juice, water, and a little bit of baby oil. Shake and spritz onto hot feet for a totally refreshing pick-me-up. The citrus will refresh and revive, and the baby oil will help moisturize.

➤ Lock the color in place with a top coat such as Seche Vite ($10; www.prosalonsupply .com), which penetrates to the base coat, forming a single, solid bond that will not discolor or yellow.

Hair Removal

Looking tanned, toned, and polished is just the first step to a successful romantic rendezvous. Making sure your skin is smooth and hair-free is your next most important step. You have plenty of ways to accomplish this very essential task.

Waxing—hot or cold wax is applied to the skin. Once it solidifies it is quickly stripped away against the direction of the growth, pulling the hair out. We like Sugar Wax Hair Removal Kit by Sally Hansen ($9.49, mass retailers). Waxing just takes a few minutes at home or in a salon. Salon prices can range from $30–$60 depending on the areas you need waxed.

Electrolysis—a very fine needle is inserted into the hair follicle, transmitting a mild electrical current designed to destroy the regenerative cells and eliminate any chance of hair growing back. Electrolysis begins at $35 a session.

Tweezing—plucking stray hairs from the root one at a time. We like the LTD Tweezer by Tweezerman ($19.99, mass retailers).

Laser treatment—a narrow beam of concentrated light is focused on a section of skin. The light destroys the hair follicles, thus preventing hair from growing back. Laser treatments cost about $60 for a session.

Hair removal meditation—a make-believe way of removing hair that we've slipped in here to see if you're paying attention. But we're sure that somewhere, someone is working on it!

Get Your Shave On!

If you think shaving is a mindless process, think and think again. Thanks to Gillette, we know a thing or two about shaving.

➤ Shower or bathe before you shave. Although women's hair is finer than men's, it is still about as tough as copper wire of the same thickness. If you hydrate hair with warm water it becomes up to 60 percent easier to cut. You can, however, soak too much, and this will cause your skin to wrinkle and swell, which means you won't be able to shave quite as close as you'd like.

➤ Wash your legs and underarms to remove natural oils and perspiration. Then, apply a generous amount of moisture-rich shave gel such as Gillette Satin Care for Women before shaving to help keep water in the hair and to ensure the razor glides easily over the skin. Soap can actually clog the razor, and many soaps cause dryness and flaking.

➤ Choose a razor that is properly equipped for the job. Gillette's Venus Vibrance with Soothing Vibrations ($10) provides a close shave and has Gillette's most advanced comfort-coated blades. It gently exfoliates to instantly reveal more radiant skin. The new Moisture Glide Strips release more lubricants per shave than any Venus cartridge for a gentle and smooth shave.

➤ Always shave with a fresh blade. Fresh blades give you a closer, smoother, and more comfortable shave and can help prevent cuts and irritation. You will probably be able to detect when your blade needs replacing if you feel a dullness or discomfort when shaving.

➤ Use a light touch when shaving, and work only in the direction that feels most comfortable. Relather before shaving the bikini and other sensitive areas.

➤ Leave the hard-to-shave spots such as ankles and the backs of knees and thighs for last.

➤ Moisturizing your legs keeps the skin hydrated and supple. When you're finished shaving, apply a rich moisturizer.

Shaving Myths

Gillette set us straight on a few old wives tales.

➤ Shaving will not make your hair grow back thicker, darker, or faster. Shaving does not affect hair growth or change the color or texture of the hair in any way.

➤ Shaving will not make your skin dry and flaky. Shaving with a razor actually helps skin look and feel smoother because the razor removes the top layer of dead skin cells.

➤ Soap and water are not all you need to get a smooth, clean shave. Shave gel actually allows the razor to glide more easily over the skin. Shave gel will not dry the skin or clog your razor the way ordinary soap will.

➤ Shaving will not remove your tan. You simply cannot shave off a tan, because tanning is a function of melanin production. Shaving actually enhances your tan by removing the flaky skin that can hide its glow.

➤ It is not a good idea to share razors with your husband or brother, because a man's hair is much coarser and damages the blade quickly. This can cause unwanted nicks and cuts. Sharing with another female will cause blade confusion; you won't necessarily be able to keep track of how much the blade is being used and when it should be changed.

➤ Shaving during the winter helps you improve the appearance of dry skin by removing that dead skin layer.

➤ You should remove underarm hair for more than cosmetic reasons. Removing underarm hair reduces the potential for bacterial buildup, which is the principal cause of underarm odor.

BIKINI BARE

We love the Personna B'kini Razor ($1) because you can get close, down there, without risking nicks or cuts from wide blades. These are small and narrow and have aloe vera and tea tree oil strips to keep you soft and moisturized while shaving. The three-pack can be found in dollar stores nationwide or at American Safety Razor Company (www.asrco.com).

Foot Creams and Lotions

We all need some good healing sole food for our feet. Here are some top picks of foot creams and lotions from our foot experts.

HIGH Benefit Bathina Sandal Scandal ($34)
www.sephora.com

You may never see your name in lights, but that doesn't mean you can't dazzle 'em with your feet. This luxurious cream is spiked with 10 percent alpha hydroxy acid, which works wonders on those dry spots. You massage it in at night, then slip your feet into the Bathina's booties and by morning your feet feel fresh, tingling, and velvety soft.

HIGH DDF Pedi-Cream ($28)
www.sephora.com

For red-carpet-worthy sashaying, DDF ups the ante with 18 percent glycolic-formulated foot cream to moisturize and soften cracked and calloused heels. They've also thrown in some spearmint and menthol to cool and refresh tired feet. It sounds like a breath mint, doesn't it?

MEDIUM Miss Oops Pedicure in a Bottle ($18)
www.missoops.com

If your local carpenter could use your feet to sand wood, then this foot cream is for you. Miss Oops exfoliates and hydrates your feet and has a non-greasy formula so you can apply it in the morning and wear your shoes without that slippery, greasy feeling. It also smells pretty, like you just had a pedicure!

LOW Pro Foot Heel Rescue Superior Moisturizing Foot Cream ($6.99)
Drugstores

Would-be cowgirls with callouses so thick and rough they could pass for a rodeo queen will find relief in this foot cream. It's a thick and rich cream for seriously dried, cracked feet. Better yet, it absorbs quickly, and there's no residue or greasy feeling for boot scootin'.

LOW Dr. Scholl's Ultra Overnight Foot Cream ($7)
Mass retailers

If you've been single for forever, it might be because of those dry, cracked heels you're sporting in bed. The entire line of Dr. Scholl's products is designed to help your feet look and feel beautiful and healthy. The Ultra Overnight Foot Cream has special moisturizers that do overtime while you're sleeping. When you wake up you'll be saying, "Hey, that sandpaper on my feet is all gone. Darn! I was going to file my nails."

THE AUTHORS' PICK is the Pro Foot. Hands down, sorry feet down, this foot cream

GILLETTE SHAVING FUN FACT
Underarm hair grows almost 50 percent faster than the hair on your legs, so shave your underarms daily for a clean feeling!

actually really and truly does get rid of dry, rough skin. We don't go anywhere without our Pro Foot!

Foot Grooming

Dr. Leslie Campbell, a member of the American Podiatric Medical Association (APMA), offers the following steps for fabulous feet:

During the winter our feet are cooped up in heavy socks and shoes and may be extra dry due to the lack of moisture in the air. In addition, the average person takes 8,000 to 10,000 steps a day. So, it's no wonder we sometimes want to take a break and treat our feet to a little pampering, especially as spring and summer approach.

In order to start the season off right, make smart choices when it comes to grooming and indulge your feet in the VIP service they deserve. The following at-home treatments, recommended by the foot experts at the APMA, will help get your feet ready to make their debut for the sexiest shoe season of the year.

Foot Preparation

➤ Fill a bucket or large basin that's big enough for your feet to soak.

➤ Find a comfortable chair where you can relax and place the bucket in front of the chair. Fill the bucket with warm water.

➤ Remove nail polish with nonacetone polish remover.

➤ Stimulate foot circulation and warm up your feet by propping one foot at a time on your lap. Grasp the foot and begin slowly moving your thumbs from the top of your toes to the bottom of your heel and back. Repeat this stroking technique as many times as needed to get your feet warmed up for some serious pampering.

➤ Use a nail clipper to cut toenails straight across. Then, use an emery board to smooth the nail edges by filing in one direction without drastically rounding the edges. When toenail edges are rounded, it increases the chances for painful ingrown toenails to develop.

Sole Relief

➤ Soak your feet in the warm water for at least 5 minutes.

➤ Raise feet out of the bucket and dip either a foot file such as Dr. Scholl's Dual-Action Swedish Foot File or a pumice stone into the water. Next, use the file or pumice stone to gently smooth the skin around the heel and the balls and sides of your feet. Stay away from a foot razor, because it removes too much skin and can easily cause an infection and permanent damage to the skin if used incorrectly. A foot file or pumice stone will do the same thing and is much less dangerous.

➤ For extra smoothing and softening, use a scrub such as Avon's Foot Works Double Action Sloughing Cream ($2.99, www.avon .com), and massage your entire foot and lower leg. The scrub exfoliates by removing dead skin buildup that is often caused by wearing certain types of shoes. Remove scrub with a damp towel.

➤ Use a fresh towel to pat feet dry and be sure to dry between each toe. While you are drying, loosen your foot joints by cupping your heel with one hand at the ankle and grabbing the top of your foot with the other. Then, rotate the foot slowly at the ankle a few times in each direction.

➤ Apply and massage a healthy amount of emollient-enriched skin lotion such as Ureacin-10 Lotion ($24.20, www.radiant skinshoppe.com), all over your feet to hydrate the skin and increase circulation. For added relief and relaxation while moisturizing, use your thumbs to apply extra pressure to the ball of your foot and arch. This will help to release tension in your arches. Then, for all-over relief, use your hand to squeeze your achilles tendon (the fleshy area above your heel), one foot at a time, for 5 seconds. Repeat two to three times.

➤ Gently push back cuticles with an instrument such as a cuticle pusher or manicure stick. Cuticles, which are located between the nail and underlying soft tissue, provide a protective barrier against infection and should never be cut. Destruction of the cuticle could result in infection, and incessantly pushing back your cuticles will only make them thicker.

Foot Finale

➤ Remove the moisturizer from your toenails and in between your toes by using soap and water. If the moisturizer remains in between your toes, it can increase the chance of a foot infection such as athlete's foot. The retained moisture also promotes nail fungus, which is a discoloration and thickening of the toenail. Pedinol's Nail Scrub ($17.99, www.beautysurg.com) helps to bleach and smooth rough, discolored, and thickened nails.

➤ Only if you have healthy nails should nail polish be applied. While it may make your toes look pretty, nail polish locks out moisture and doesn't allow the nail or nail bed to breathe, so people who suffer from already discolored toenails will aggravate their condition by not allowing their nails to be exposed to the air. Whether you have discolored nails or not, it is advisable to remove polish regularly.

➤ Before bed, very lightly wrap cellophane around your entire foot. The cellophane will act as a makeshift sauna by locking in moisture. By morning your feet will feel soothingly soft.

➤ Continue to keep your feet healthy all season long by protecting the skin that surrounds them with a waterproof, oil-free sunscreen every time you slip on your favorite pair of sandals or go barefoot at the beach.

Beauty Time Warp

Do you remember Body on Tap and Gee Your Hair Smells Terrific shampoo? How about Lifebuoy soap, Tangee lipstick, or even *Pssssst* instant shampoo? After much digging we found that you can still purchase these old classics in their original formulations. The Vermont Country Store (www.vermontcountry store.com) carries lots of golden oldies that will recapture a time in your life with hard-to-find products you thought were discontinued. "We capture the emotional connection of *'Hey, I remember that!'* and our nostalgic products generate familiarity for our customers," says Cindy Marshall, director of marketing for The Vermont Country Store. Here's what we found there:

Tangee lipstick and Tangee rouge
(each $12.95)

Tangee was a cosmetics company, started by George W. Luft in New York City in the 1930s. Constance Luft Huhn created the world's number one lipstick. The name *Tangee* is short for tangerine, one of the most popular lipstick colors from the 40s and the actual color of Tangee lipstick. Tangee was very popular with the socialites in New York and the very chic Hollywood stars from the 30s because although each Tangee lipstick is tangerine, it changes color, depending on the pigment in your skin, to a deeper tangerine, soft pink, or raspberry. One advertisement from 1947 read, "So, why not join all of the beautiful ladies of Hollywood—why not join the best dressed, the most attractive women of the world and glamorize yourself with Tangee—the world's No. 1 lipstick, regardless of price." From a 1940s advertisement for Tangee lipstick titled *War, Women and Lipstick*: "For the first time in history, women-power is a factor in war. Millions of you are fighting and working side by side with your men. It's a reflection of the free democratic way of life that you have succeeded in keeping your femininity, even though you are doing a man's work. No lipstick—ours or anyone else's—will win the war, but it symbolizes one of the reasons why we are fighting . . . the precious right of women to be feminine and lovely under any circumstances."

Psssssst Instant Shampoo ($11.95)

This product cleans your hair without water—just spray and brush! Clairol introduced it to the market in 1967, and it was the first of its kind.

Lifebuoy Soap ($9.90)

First introduced in 1894 by Lever Brothers in Liverpool, England, Lifebuoy was an affordable soap for personal hygiene. It became a big hit in the United States after Lifebuoy soap introduced American radio audiences to a new concept and created a new phrase in the English language—B.O. Worried about the effects of "nervous B.O."—not finding romance or missing out on the big promotion—Americans began to bathe more frequently, and Lifebuoy became a bestselling soap in the country.

Tired Old Ass Soak ($14.95)

Ok, this isn't a golden oldie, but we couldn't resist the name. It's a blend of salts high in iron and trace minerals and 100 percent pure essential oils of rosemary, eucalyptus, and vetiver, among others. Tired Old Ass Soak perks you up again in a way that is no joke. If you're too pressed for time to take a bath, take a footbath—or quit your job. Life is too short to be worn out. Biodegradable, planet friendly, and 100 percent natural, it's a perfect gift for all the tired old bodies you know.

Gee Your Hair Smells Terrific ($9.90)

This shampoo is a 70s icon. It has a flowery and spicy scent in a groovy pink or blue bottle, and you can buy it in the same formula you remember at www.geeyourhairsmellsterrific.com.

Body on Tap shampoo and conditioner ($8.75)

This is another 70s beauty icon. The only source for this product appears to be www .outofafricatrading.com.

The Attractive Apocrypha

There are important materials that go with every Buyble, Beauty or otherwise, other stories that just didn't fit this time around. The *Beauty Buyble* is intended to focus on beauty products to bring out the internal Goddess in you (therefore inspiring "Venus Envy"—the jealousy felt by non-*Beauty Buyble* Babes toward the enlightened readers of this hallowed tome).

No, all *Beauty Buyble* Babes also need to pay attention to fashion flourishes that enhance your newly found awesomeness. For example, why wear just a plain old headset when on the phone, at home or the office, presumably to keep your hands free while applying your new-found favorite products? A *Beauty Buyble* Babe might show a little flash by wearing a Swapset (www.swapsets.com)—a chicly customized telephone headset, complete with colorful headband, headphone or headset, and a number of shiny dangles. Or perhaps a funky new handbag like a Junior Drake bag, because *Beauty Buyble* Babes like to keep it classy, but still want a little edge. Where do Halle Berry, Geena Davis, Queen Latifah, Tyra Banks, Sharon Stone, and Kelly Ripa hide their beauty products? Answer: their Junior Drake bag! Visit www.juniordrake .com for retailers near you.

Sound like shameless plugs? Well, they are and they aren't. We love these products, and these are just a few examples of what the *Beauty Buyble* Babes crave—the fun and the funky; the agony and the ecstasy. It is all part of beauty's rich tapestry and we encourage all *Beauty Buyble* Babes to explore their fashion world. There are just three rules: 1) No stockings with open-toed sandals, 2) Burn all scrunchies, 3) Stay clear of Spandex. Let us know what you find!

Afterword

Being a *Beauty Buyble* girl is more than just looking runway fabulous at all times. Certainly, we'd like you to do that, but realistically we know that won't happen, so we here at the *BB* will settle for you just looking and feeling your absolute best. Even D-listers need flawless skin, luscious locks, and party-perfect makeovers. We think of *The Beauty Buyble* as the beauty insider in your back pocket, here to help you ditch your old products for a set of new, shiny ones and be on your way to a newfound addiction—you! So get out of the beauty ghetto and make peace with the fact that you are beautiful, and with some hope and a little sarcasm along the way we'll turn you into a bonafide *Beauty Buyble* Babe in no time.

If you like what you've read, please let us know. If you're not completely enchanted by this book, please do not try to contact us in any way. We don't want to be shushed, and we don't want to hear your criticism of our witticism.

Beautifully yours,
Paula and Maureen,
the *Beauty Buyble* Babes

Acknowledgments

To the BEAutiful staff at ReganBooks, our publisher **Judith Regan** for Buying the beauty BUYble and always thinking outside the box with us; Thank you for the amazing opportunity. Our editor **Cassie Jones,** your commitment, talent and dedication deserve an award, **Tammie Guthrie,** for unwavering organization and support, **Jessica Di Biase,** for picking up where Tammie left off; **Jennifer Brunn** and **Amy Franklin** for tremendous publicity efforts; **Lauren Rouleau** for great goodie bags and marketing; **Adrienne Makowski, Kurt Andrews, Leah Ho,** and **Kris Tobiassen** for tremendous design and production efforts; **Maggie Bullock** for sitting through a long lecture about her eggs while providing lots and lots of expert advice for the book; **Anne Hardy, Scott Vincent Borba, Dan Feldman,** and **Katherine Hickland** for joining us in the very beginning; **Doreen Gillis** for camera-ready makeup, **Joshua Farrington** for amazing hair; **Thomas Card** for gorgeous photography; **Cara Birnbaum** for helping us while working on her own book; **Mark Garrison** for his unyielding generosity, great hair, great tips and a great attitude; **Lorri Goddard-Clark** for the best hair coloring tips; **Think PR** for being on the ball at all times; **Tasha Turner** for making sure that the woman of color was well represented in this book; to **Eden Grimaldi** of Media Craft for just plain getting it; to **Mary Wenger** for corralling publicists and products; to **Amy McCloskey** for helping us on all fronts in exchange for beauty products; to **Brooke Bryant** at Cloutier and **Peter Ashworth** for jumping in at the last minute; to **Allison Slater** at Sephora and **Adam Gerstein** with Beauty Addicts for teaming up with us and **Margaret Jaworski** for her genius creativity.

From Paula

To my mother **Mary Wenger** for teaching me how to be and feel beautiful, inside and out, and for so many things she did to help us get this book off the ground that are too numerous to list; **Maureen Regan**, my friend, coauthor and the person who truly made this all possible, and thus changed the course of my life forever; **Judith Regan** for giving me my first book opportunity; **Stephen Silverman** for making me feel like I could accomplish anything when I was his student at Columbia; to **Delores Mills** for so lovingly taking care of me and my family whenever we need her; and most importantly to my husband **John Conway** for loving me unconditionally and allowing me to fill our home with piles of pretty products while I was writing this book.

xo Paula

From Maureen

Rita Regan for teaching me about natural beauty, **Leo Regan** for passing on his high cheeks bones, **Judith Regan** for teaching me how to "get over it," **Patty** and **Michelle Madonna** for being so beautiful, **Marc Libarle** for unwavering friendship and guidance, **Caroline Larrouilh**, for giving me my first red lipstick, **Dee Dee Liestenfeltz** for beautiful friendship, **Cynthia Robins**, a great teacher of beauty and style, **Cynthia Cooper**, product junkie extraordinaire, thanks for always sharing, **Maribel Ortiz** and her family for loving Ava as much as I do. My dear friend and coauthor **Paula Conway** who's generosity, love, talent, and beauty has changed my life forever.

To my husband **Will Dunkak**, and children **Quinn** and **Ava**, who always make me radiate from within. I love you.

xo Maureen

To our *Beauty Buyble* experts: Gina Bertolliti, Oscar Blandi, Trae Bodge, Scott Vincent Borba, Kathleen Burke, Karla Cay, Chip Cordelli, Christo, Dr. Leslie Copeland, Dr. Doris Day, Richard Dean, Eliza, Dr. Jeffrey Epstein, Gordon Elliott, Dan Feldman, Mark Garrison, Dr. Michael Ghalili, Dr. Dennis Gross, Katherine Hickland, Sally Hershberger, Brad Johns, David H. Kingsley Ph.D., Reiko Kobayashi, Ellin Lavar, Dr. Diane C. Madfres, Lorraine Massey, Dr. Philip Miller, Georgette Mosbacher, Ouidad,

Orlando Pita, Rebecca Restrepo, Edita Robertson, Mally Roncal, Dr. Neil Sadick, Eva Scrivo, Claudia Shaum, Jacqueline Shepherd, Troy Surratt, David Tippie, Tasha Turner, Robert Vettica, Jennifer Urezzio, Rita Utkis, Steve Vu, Kyle White, Careth Whitchurch and Rachel Whitehurst.

Finally, we'd like to thank our league of intrepid testers: Caroline Larrouilh, Dee Dee Liestenfeltz, Michelle Madonna, Rita Regan, Patty Regan, Maribel Ortiz, Christine Onorati, Therese Gamba, Cynthia Robins, Terri Catania, Carolyn Catania, Cynthia Cooper, Toni Johnson, Gwen Garrett, Coimbra Sirica, Barbara O'Neill, Brittany Attardi, Julie Vargo, Sandy Dupkas, Rosey Livering, Ava Dunkak and Quinn Dunkak, Elizabeth Ciresi, Anne Hardy, Maggie Bullock, Suz Amedi, Pat Hagan, Terri Hoornstra, J. P. Hoornstra, Shammy, Jean Copeland, Doris Herndon, Debbie Kuban, Delores Mills, Irving Mills, Karen Giunta, Cara Birnbaum, Patricia Land, Mary Wenger, Leslie Copeland, Debbie Kuban, Jennifer Kuban, Lisa Davis, Nancy Hirsch.

Notes

Notes

Notes